Basic Psychiatric Concepts in Nursing

BASIC PSYCHIATRIC CONCEPTS IN NURSING

Third Edition

Joan J. Kyes, R.N., M.S.N.

Chief Psychiatric Nurse
Altoona Hospital Community Mental Health Center, Pa.
Clinical Nurse Consultant
Hollidaysburg State Hospital and Leech Farms Veterans Hospital
Lecturer in Continuing Education
Pennsylvania State University
formerly Clinical Specialist in Psychiatric Nursing
Hollidaysburg State Hospital, Pa.

Charles K. Hofling, M.D.

Professor of Psychiatry
Department of Neurology and Psychiatry
College of Medicine
St. Louis University
Visiting Professor of Psychiatry
College of Medicine
University of Cincinnati

J. B. LIPPINCOTT COMPANY
Philadelphia   Toronto

Distributed in Great Britain by
Blackwell Scientific Publications
London   Oxford   Edinburgh

ISBN-0-397-54153-8

Library of Congress Catalog Card Number 74-2370

Printed in the United States of America

2 4 6 8 9 7 5 3

Library of Congress Cataloging in Publication Data

Kyes, Joan J.
    Basic psychiatric concepts in nursing.

    Includes bibliographies.
    1. Psychiatric nursing. 2. Psychiatry. I. Hofling, Charles K., joint author. II. Title.
    [DNLM: 1. Psychiatric nursing. 2. Psychiatry—Nursing texts.
WY160 K99b 1974]
RC440.K9   1974   616.8′9′0023613   74-2370
ISBN 0-397-54153-8

PREFACE

All areas of nursing practice are entering what promises to be one of the most exciting, most fruitful, and most rewarding periods in the history of nursing. There is the stimulus of new knowledge relating to physical and emotional aspects of the human condition. Understanding and assimilation of this knowledge by nurses, demonstrated through competent clinical practice, has resulted in the increasing recognition of the role of the nurse in the delivery of health care.

The increased responsibility of today's practitioner has prompted us to prepare a thorough revision of *Basic Psychiatric Concepts in Nursing*. We have, in this third edition, placed the emphasis on the practice of nursing and the presentation of nursing care material which will help the student to move from the theoretical to the operational level. We have preserved the clear description of psychiatric theory from the previous editions and explained and demonstrated through case examples how the nurse can intervene. We have put the focus on the dynamics of the nurse's role and function. We have stressed the importance of psychiatric concepts in all areas of nursing practice and the necessity of making these concepts a vital part of the nurse's daily life-style.

As in the earlier editions of this textbook, we are writing primarily for the undergraduate student of nursing, yet with sufficient attention to detail of both theory and practice so that the material will be of real value to the advanced student in psychiatry as well. At a time when nurse practitioners are being recognized as performing with some independence, when state laws are being studied and altered to permit the expansion of the role and function of the nurse, and when the American Nurses' Association is moving toward developing means by which excellence in the practice of nursing will be recognized through certification of the nurse practitioner, it is increasingly important that students in all levels of nursing education familiarize themselves both with theory and its practical application to the direct care of patients.

Topics of increasing concern to nursing have been extensively rewritten. These include drug abuse, problems of sexual deviation, the understanding of behavior, developing a sensitivity to the human condition, nursing management of the neurotic and psychotic patient, the understanding of self in relation to interpersonal interactions with peers, supervisors, subordinates and patient, and the recognition of common emotional problems faced by all hospitalized patients who, in their efforts to adjust to and understand the sterile, frightening and oft-times unfeeling atmosphere of the hospital environment, become critically overwhelmed.

We gratefully acknowledge the help and inspiration of Madeleine M. Leininger, R.N., M.S.N., Ph.D. to earlier editions of this book.

JOAN J. KYES
CHARLES K. HOFLING

CONTENTS

1

Applying Psychiatric Concepts to Nursing Practice

All Behavior Has Meaning * Developing Sensitivity to the
Human Condition * Fundamental Psychiatric Concepts

To be a therapeutic factor in the care of patients, the nurse needs to have knowledge about people, their needs and feelings, and their ways of expressing them. She needs to understand behavior in herself, in the patient, in his family and friends, and the impact this behavior has on the care of the patient, or perhaps on the outcome of his illness.

Nurses find themselves with various feelings or attitudes as they relate with and care for patients. A patient who is demanding or whining may cause the nurse to visit him briefly, to prohibit him from expressing his feelings, or to assign less trained individuals to wait upon him. She may find she has difficulty ministering to a patient with an incurable disease or staying with one who is suffering a great deal or dying. After all, she entered nursing to cure people, and incurable patients do not lend themselves to this image.

Nurses who understand behavior recognize that the patient who demands that tasks be performed for him (such as winding his bed up or down, putting the window up or down, wanting his back rubbed, his pillow fluffed, or fresh water) is really saying that he is anxious or frightened and wants someone near him. He is distressed and concerned and unable to work out the anxieties resulting from his illness. When the nurse understands this behavior, she is more able to respond by meeting the patient's needs rather than by withdrawing from his excessive demands. She can allow herself to explore with the patient what he is really trying to say, or what his behavior really indicates.

The experienced nurse knows that a relatively simple routine such as the bath can become a valuable vehicle for communication between nurse and patient. The few minutes required for the administration of a medication can be made useful to the patient if the nurse is skillful in observing, listening, and responding to cues. As the nurse becomes more knowledgeable about psychiatric concepts and more adept in applying this knowledge at the patient care level, she will discover that she can use herself quite skillfully through her relationship with the patient and will no longer need a task as a security measure in relating to him. This nurse will be able to approach the patient before he calls, secure in her ability to relate with him, to identify his needs, and to meet them. She will no longer fear "being taken advantage of" or become exhausted by the many unmet needs around her.

In the last analysis, there is very little basis for the often heard excuse of "no time." There is not so much a shortage of *nurses* as there is a shortage of *nursing*. Understanding the meaning of behavior and acquiring skills in the therapeutic use of oneself are means by which the nurse can be purposefully useful to the patient. Nursing provides an opportunity for giving care which considers man as a whole being. Mind and body are not separated, so that incidents that affect one part affect the other. This holistic view of the personality is significant to any examination of man's reaction to stress or strain. One of the hazards of medicine and nursing is that prolonged exposure to many sick people and familiarity with hospitals often blind nurses and doctors to the emotional impact these circumstances have on the patient. Health care personnel tend to forget (unless they, themselves, or members of their family are hospitalized) that experiences which to them are matters of daily routine, could well be viewed by the patient as awesome and frightening.

ALL BEHAVIOR HAS MEANING

All behavior serves a purpose, and can be understood and modified. Through behavior, human beings express their physical, psychological, social, and spiritual needs. The extent to which these needs may be identified varies from person to person and from time to time. Needs can be described in terms of developmental levels. That is, they can range from infantile, primitive levels upward toward maturity. The nurse must determine the area of greatest need in the patient based on her observation of him—his actions, conversation, and appearance. Her ability to recognize these needs and to respond to them therapeutically depends on her own basic knowledge of human behavior, the degree to which she can accept the behavior demonstrated by others, and the degree of security with which she is able to look at her own behavior.

Staff members have the same needs as patients and can give to patients only as their own needs are met. Nurses and nursing students can respond to a patient's need for control if they feel safe and certain that their supervisors or clinical instructors will help and support them as they give care. They can give the patient freedom to develop his own resources when they, in turn, feel the freedom to develop theirs. Inherent in this, for both patient and nurse, is the "right to fail." Carefully made plans do not always come to successful ends. Both patients and nurses need the freedom to make mistakes as they work together to resolve the problems of living with illness. This point needs further elaboration.

Through objective and thoughtful evaluations of ongoing practices, nurses gain valuable insight into the outcome of their professional behavior and learn about areas in which these behaviors may need to be altered, restructured, or discontinued. When this occurs, the nurse, whose practice has been evaluated, must consciously consider how she views the result of this study. Does she accept the challenge to find new, innovative ways to solve patient care problems, or does she consider her practice in these areas a mistake or an error for which she must make atonement?

Traditionally, many nurses and nursing students were taught, or came to believe, that in the practice of nursing, mistakes and errors could not be tolerated. Those who subscribe to this belief tend to judge their practice and that of others exclusively in terms of either "right or wrong," "good or bad." Consequently, it becomes increasingly more difficult for them to evaluate their services to patients, because evaluations frequently signify areas of needed change which the practitioners perceive as indications that some mistake or error had occurred.

Right and good in terms of nursing practice mean that the patient appears to respond favorably to nursing care and treatment, and that the practitioners carry out the physician's orders, nursing procedures, and hospital policies in a precise way, demonstrating by tangible, onsite evidence, that all "nursing tasks" are completed by the end of their shift. Conversely, wrong and bad mean that the patient does not appear to be responding to nursing care and treatment, that medications may have been late, that nursing procedures and housekeeping chores are not completed before the physician's or supervisor's early rounds, and that oncoming shifts are faced with harried staff, unkempt linen closets, messy treatment rooms, and nurses' stations piled high with incomplete charts and paper work.

It is no wonder that nurses in this type of situation feel professionally inadequate and overwhelmed, and are unable to assess the situation honestly, to examine their own feelings and behavior, and to look objectively at what might be occurring with the patient. To do so, with the philosophy just described, would be to admit to mistakes and errors in terms of good nursing practice. Therefore, these nurses are unable to work through their feelings and do not grow to new levels of competency.

Nurses who do not view the results of evaluations as indications of "practice failures" and who have supervisors and/or clinical specialists to assist and support them in developing their own resources, grow more professionally competent and personally secure. This requires an attitude free from threat, which allows nurses to approach the solving of patient care problems from a dynamic orientation and which permits them to be comfortable enough to expose their practice for assessment and evaluation by others. In this context, the word *dynamic* refers to the forces governing behavior. Looking for the reasons behind a person's behavior and examining the forces operating in the situation constitute the dynamic approach to nursing. The following anecdote is a simplified illustration of this principle.

At bedtime, Mrs. F. began to request from the nursing student many varied and apparently unnecessary attentions. Each request made a trip to Mrs. F.'s room necessary. The student became more and more bothered by these "interruptions," but she continued to answer the requests as quickly as possible, with as little time investment as possible.

One night, after the student had hurried in and out of the room several times, Mrs. F. became very angry and was so demanding that the student refused to answer her signal again. At this point the student sought help from her instructor. Together they began to analyze the situation to find out the "whys" of Mrs. F.'s behavior and the "whys" of the student's responses, thus uncovering some of the dynamic forces that were in operation.

In talking with Mrs. F. the student discovered that she was afraid to go to sleep because she thought she might die and wanted someone near. Her requests were unnecessary in terms of the articles wanted, but they were the patient's only known way of asking the nurse to stay. The student, feeling burdened by the pressing responsibility of other patients, had neither taken the time nor thought to observe and listen to Mrs. F., and had in effect ignored the obvious plea that was being made. As Mrs. F. became more frightened, lonely, and desperate for reassurance, she became more insistent. The student, in the same measure, became more resistant and denying, and communication was stalemated.

The dynamic nursing approach insists that the nurse search continually for the why of behavior. She must ask herself what the behavior is saying, what it is asking for, and what the appropriate nursing response is. This means that there is no routine patient and no routine care. The nurse is always planning care for a particular patient, with particular problems and needs, in a particular situation.

Dynamic nursing does not in any way lessen the nurse's responsibility for understanding the nature and treatment of disease. It adds a new dimension for creativity and satisfaction in professional nursing.

Managing one's own feelings while dealing with a patient's feelings requires professional skill. Through the understanding of psychiatric concepts and their application to the therapeutic care of patients, nurses are more able to help themselves and others deal with the multiplicity of feelings which arise in the daily task of living. Personal problems and feelings may conflict seriously with a nurse's desire to be helpful to the patient, and she may not understand why she behaved as she did. The following situation illustrates how a nurse's feelings interfered with helping a patient.

Miss B., the nurse, was concerned about her patient who was very sad, had no visitors, and was frequently seen crying in her pillow. When approached, the patient often said, "No one really understands what is happening to me and no one cares." Miss B. spent considerable time sitting with the patient and listening, but found herself becoming more and more irritated. One day the head nurse overheard Miss B. saying in an exasperated way, "I know how you feel; I'm lonely here too, but I'm not crying."

When Miss B. and the head nurse explored the situation, it became clear that Miss B. found she had feelings very like those the patient was trying to express. As she listened to the patient, she found herself joining in the sadness and loneliness. This made the nurse feel more and more helpless and eventually angry. By discussing her feelings with the head nurse, Miss B. was able to recognize them so that she could then reexamine the patient's problems and help her deal more realistically with them.

Nurses and nursing students need to be reassured that in the process of dealing with people, negative feelings, such as anger, do arise and are normal. Feelings are not under conscious control, but for the most part the action or behavior which follows the feelings can be controlled. This requires the nurse to have some understanding of human behavior and a willingness to identify and explore her negative feelings with those who may help her. However, nurses who believe that negative feelings are not legitimate in the interpersonal situation deny their own human condition, and tend to block healthy exploration of feelings in others. This attitude extends itself beyond the patient into interpersonal relationships with supervisors, instructors, physicians, subordinates, and peers. Situations should be fostered which promote open relationships between all concerned. Negative situations which are resolved free more effort for the task of caring for patients.

Patients' visitors have long been a source of ambivalent feelings for nurses. Some view visitors as a "curse" in that they always seem to be in the way, while others find them useful in assisting with feedings, answering minor requests for the patient, or entertaining him. For the most part this attitude depends upon the age of the patient, the amount of professional nursing care he requires, and how demanding he and his visitors are of the nurse's time. Many nurses fail to recognize that the patient's family and friends have a great deal of influence upon him, and that their sense of well-being is important if they are to help the patient feel secure. People who are significant to the patient support him in his time of sickness or distress.

The nurse who feels that visitors are an "unnecessary evil" which she must tolerate in the course of her duty, tends to ignore them, to relate infrequently with them, or even to indicate that they are interfering with her care of the patient. Even if it is not stated verbally, visitors feel uncomfortable because they pick up this attitude and feeling in the nurse. When visitors are uncomfortable, patients feel uncomfortable and anxious. They look forward to visitors because it breaks up the monotony of the day and indicates that someone is concerned about them. The nurse who takes a few minutes to show understanding of and concern for the feeling of "those who are concerned about the patient," will find that her patients respond more positively to her care.

Members of the public who visit the hospitalized patient carry their impressions of hospital staff and their care of the patient back with them into the community. A nurse who is insensitive to the feelings of visitors contributes to the negative feelings the community may have of the hospital and the kind of care one receives there. This may override all of the good care she has assisted with in terms of the patient. The nurse who extends her understanding of basic human needs beyond the patient to his friends and family contributes even more to the patient's feeling of trust in her. Family members or significant friends need to feel involved. Allowing them to assist by reassuring the patient or by supporting him in decisions that he must make is more important than giving them the feeling that they are intruding or not needed.

DEVELOPING SENSITIVITY TO THE HUMAN CONDITION

Members of the health care professions must constantly remind themselves that patients are people with certain rights. It is very dehumanizing to find oneself no longer able to control or to make simple basic decisions about the personal daily events in one's life. It is both frightening and embarrassing to realize that one has become helpless and in many ways quite dependent on others in order to have one's basic human needs met. Nurses must be sensitive to what is happening to the patient and in as many ways as possible help to preserve his dignity and rights.

When people move into hospitals, their territory or range of control becomes greatly limited in relation to that to which they are usually accustomed. Depending on the type of accommodations which are available, or which they can afford, this could consist of a private room with bath, a room shared with one other person, or a wardlike area ranging from three to thirty patients or more. Frequently, patients can claim only the space around their beds as theirs. The manner in which the nurse approaches this space can be interpreted by the patient as either trespassing or respect for his domain. Frequently, without the patient's permission, nurses begin to search through bureau drawers and night stands, looking for linen hidden by other nurses, bodycare lotion, and so on; toss someone else's soiled linen on the patient's chair, or enter the room without speaking and remove articles or objects from it. This behavior makes the patient feel that he is an insignificant being or perhaps an unwelcomed visitor in a house which belongs solely to the members of the health care professions. It is important for nurses to consider ways to preserve the patient's privacy, dignity, and freedom of decision in as many ways as possible. This assures the patient that nursing staff members are interested in his personal well-being and his returning to an independent state as soon as possible.

Nurses need to understand dependency and all of its manifestations in order to plan more clearly the best treatment for the patient. Modern psychological medicine accepts and recognizes the fact that a sick person becomes a somewhat dependent individual because this is one of the ways each person first reacts to injury, sickness, or pain. In acute phases of illness, the patient's interests become more centered on what is happening to him than they do when he is well. We see this clearly in a child who is acutely ill. Except for a soft, cuddly toy, he seems to lose his usual interest in toys and playmates, is pleased to see his parents but does not have the energy to inquire about happenings at home, and narrows his interests to his immediate discomfort and those who are directly treating or caring for him.

Adult patients react similarly, with some readily accepting the fact that they are ill and need to be in a passive, dependent position. To these patients, illness may be welcomed, inasmuch as it allows them to depend upon others, giving them relief from the trials and responsibilities that they have been facing. Others find illness more difficult to accept. These patients may deny their illness and dependency, for to them illness usually means a loss of self-esteem and status, a personal affront which makes remaining in bed synonymous with being a weakling. At times it is frightening and almost intolerable to learn that one must rely partially or completely upon another for intimate, physical care. Many adults have been accustomed to attending to their own personal needs for a long period of time. Being helpless, even for a brief period or in a limited sense, has a tremendous impact upon them.

Some nurses may encourage dependency in patients by doing many things for them. Others interpret dependency somewhat differently and tend to encourage patients to be independent earlier in an illness. These nurses often view dependency as a negative aspect of illness and frequently deny obvious signs of it. To them dependency in adult patients is viewed as an inadequacy and the ensuing behavior, manipulative and controlling. They charge patients to "act their age" and react with disgust toward those whose efforts to have basic needs met manifest themselves at a less mature level.

A helpless, regressed, and dependent patient may mean to the nurse that she is a failure, and she may feel that something drastic or unfavorable has happened to him. Occasionally, the one who treats the patient at the dependent level may be reprimanded and told to treat him as an adult at all times. A patient may be chronologically an adult; however, illness can shift his emotional age so that he may be acting considerably younger. Respect for him means accepting him and meeting his needs at the moment, recognizing that healthy independence emerges from healthy dependency.

Dependency upon others is a fundamental human need, both during the early developmental periods of life and in any critical and stressful period. Nurses who have difficulty accepting dependency in others can do nothing but harm to those who require permission to be dependent during the critical times of their lives. One of the wonderful things about the human condition is interdependency and the need for sharing with other human beings. It is a tremendous disservice to the patient when staff communicates to him that it is wrong for him to have feelings of dependency or to exhibit behavior which indicates that certain regressive needs must be met. Those who have never quite worked through their own dependency needs will frequently punish others for similar feelings. Often subordinate nursing personnel may compete with the patients for the nurse's attention. Nurses also demonstrate dependency needs when they require constant reassurance from their supervisors or are unable to express what they need to say without a great deal of support from other members of the team. Until nurses and others in the health care professions are able to face their own feelings about dependency or to have some recognition of their own dependency needs, they will not be free to interact with or to support the patient at the level his needs demand.

Those preparing themselves for professional nursing practice need to explore their own personal views and philosophies about dependency. Some people enter the health care professions because of a strong desire to be needed, in a helping way, by other human beings. These people may tend to foster dependency in the patient and, in a sense, communicate to him that being dependent and in need is good patient behavior. Patients are frequently placed in situations where they are completely helpless and must depend entirely upon others to meet their needs. Initially, these patients may feel helpless and inadequate because of their inability to care for themselves, but grow to accept their dependency because it may unconsciously be reinforced by staff. The patient, in a subtle way, gets the message, "If you get too well or too independent, we will throw you out of the hospital."

Independence grows out of dependency. Man has a natural tendency to move toward increasing degrees of independence. The individuals striving for personal freedom, or independence, can be observed from early childhood until the advanced years of life. The nurse will find it important to recognize those moments when a patient can *realistically* and *appropriately* be independent. By her recognition and support of these strivings, the nurse will help him increase his confidence and personal satisfactions. Some patients need considerable time and patience before they can make independent decisions and assume responsibilities, both of which can be therapeutic steps in their rehabilitation. Time must be allowed for patients to achieve these goals.

THE APPRECIATION OF FUNDAMENTAL PSYCHIATRIC CONCEPTS AS A PREREQUISITE TO THE DEVELOPMENT OF GOOD PROFESSIONAL NURSING PRACTICE

Growth in understanding people's behavior from the simple or obvious forms to the more obscure and complex is one of the major tasks that the nursing student faces and accomplishes in her education. The physical aspects of nursing care receive appreciable attention, and nurses feel generally comfortable and competent while attending to the relatively easily determined physical needs of the patient. Recognition of his emotional needs or problems is no more or less important, but it is certainly more difficult. The psychological and human relationship concepts are woven into all aspects of nursing, and neglect of these will be a deterrent in the patient's progress toward recovery. Emotional problems have significant effects on the physical conditions of the body. The disease from which the patient is suffering, family problems, hospital tensions, and many other environmental factors may combine to overwhelm him.

As the nurse cares for a patient, she can learn relatively quickly to recognize the more obvious emotional difficulties. The patient who weeps, who cannot agree to treatment, or who cannot allow himself to remain in the hospital is showing very open signs of distress. It requires the most thoughtful and diligent use of intelligence and knowledge for the nurse to begin to understand the meaning of the behavior and to respond to it in ways that will allow the patient to work at his problem in a more mature manner. If the nurse responds to a patient as she would in an ordinary social situation, she is neglecting to fulfill her role as a therapeutic member of the treatment team.

Today, there persists a tendency to assume that "common sense" and "good will" constitute adequate preparation for therapeutic, professional handling of the nurse-patient relationship. It is usually conceded that a few technics are needed for dealing with specific, trying situations along with a certain amount of clinical experience. In addition, the hope is often expressed that nurses and nursing students will use a certain amount of intuition. Exactly how one arrives at the technic, how one best utilizes clinical experience, and how intuition is deepened and expanded, often remain quite obscure. Such vagueness sometimes accompanies the evaluation of the effectiveness of the nurse-patient relationship when one is not quite sure what to expect from the relationship as part of the overall treatment program. It is extremely easy to ignore certain outcomes that are actually therapeutic failures and to be uncertain as to where credit belongs with certain favorable results.

The following case study illustrates several aspects of this discussion. It deals with a hospital situation that is so frequent that it appears to be almost commonplace: obtaining permission to operate. Yet the situation is a complex one, full of drama. Notice that in this instance, as in many like it, the handling of the patient, not the patient's lesion alone, becomes a life-and-death matter, although this aspect of the situation could have been rationalized.

Notice, too, in reading the first part of the study, those points where a number has been inserted in parentheses. At such points, the responses of the nurse (not only what she said and did, but also what she thought to herself) have temporarily been deleted. The student is asked to consider how she might evaluate the situation at these points and what she might say and do. In particular, consider how far one might effectively go, equipped with common sense and good intentions alone.

Case 1-1

Mrs. C. W. was a patient on a large women's surgical ward at a general hospital. She had been admitted for diagnostic evaluation. She was a quiet, attractive, and dignified woman in her early forties.

Miss R., an afternoon staff nurse on the ward, was working with Mrs. C. W. and found her an exceptionally easy patient to care for. Mrs. C. W. was ambulatory, and she not only performed readily all the aspects of personal hygiene expected of her but went beyond this in being helpful to other patients. Miss R. rather liked the patient, but found her difficult to know. Although Mrs. C. W. seemed to appreciate the nurse's interest, she was quite reserved in conversation, occasionally concealing various minor discomforts and inconveniences. Miss R. felt that her patient was also trying to conceal a great deal of tension beneath her polite, composed exterior.

During the diagnostic period, Mrs. C. W. was visited twice by her husband and her pretty teenage daughter. Nurse R. noted that in the daughter's presence the patient strove to maintain an appearance of relaxed good humor.

After several days, a diagnosis was reached. Miss R. learned from the head nurse that the surgical resident and the intern had taken the patient aside during morning rounds and told her that she had cancer of the bowel. Mrs. C. W. had seemed to be seriously affected by the news, but had said very little. The resident had gone on to tell her that the condition was operable, that there was no evidence of spread of the tumor, and that her chances of recovery were good. The operation proposed would involve resection of the neoplasm and the adjacent bowel, and the construction of an ileostomy.

That afternoon, when ward activity was at a minimum, Mrs. C. W. approached Nurse R. and asked about the exact nature of her disease and the details of the proposed operation. (1)

In the course of the conversation, she referred to her mother, now dead for some years, whom she had nursed through a lingering final illness, during which the mother had been confined to bed with a stroke. Somehow the patient's reference to her mother appeared to have more significance than the mere parallel between two serious illnesses would explain. (2)

That evening, during the visiting hour, Mrs. C. W.'s husband and her daughter came to see her. From snatches of conversation that were overheard and from the demeanor of the visitors, Miss R. received the surprising impression that Mrs. C. W. was not disclosing the diagnosis and the proposal of operation. Later, at bedtime, Miss R. had the opportunity to ask the patient casually about the visit. After some preliminary remarks, Mrs. C. W. said, "You know, I didn't tell them the bad news. I want to know more about it. They have lots on their minds, too. My husband works awfully hard to provide a living for us. He's at that filling station 12 hours a day—sometimes more. And Louise [the daughter] is so young. She's smart, and pretty too. Has her head full of the boys. She's going to a party tonight. She's the most popular girl on our block." (3)

When she came on duty the following day, Nurse R. looked at Mrs. C. W.'s chart. There was a short note, describing the staff surgeon's visit and stating that he agreed fully with the resident's diagnosis and treatment recommendations. The note ended with the words: "The procedure was then explained to the patient, *but she refused operation.*"

While Miss R. was looking at Mrs. C. W.'s chart, the surgical resident came over to the nurses' station to write some orders for the next day. The nurse and the doctor began speaking about Mrs. C. W. The resident stressed the patient's "unreasonableness," in contrast with her intelligently cooperative behavior throughout the diagnostic period. Actually, the only semblance of a reason Mrs. C. W. had given in connection with her refusal of operation had been her doubts that the procedure would be successful. (4)

After some further conversation (to be described shortly), the resident decided to request a psychiatric consultation for Mrs. C. W. He asked the nurse to acquaint the patient with this step.

Miss R. went to Mrs. C. W., who was sitting beside her bed, pretending to look at a magazine. The patient had been crying. At the sight of the nurse, her lips tightened, but she greeted Miss R. politely. (5)

The situation up to this point may be summarized as follows: An intelligent, "cooperative," and rational patient has been found to have a potentially fatal disease. An approved treatment for the disease exists, offering a reasonable chance of saving the patient's life. While a serious procedure, the operation itself does not involve a grave mortality risk. Although the patient is fairly young, has a good husband and an attractive child, and, apart from the illness, does not appear to be under exceptional environmental stress, she refuses the potentially lifesaving operation. She does so even though the doctors have been sincere, frank, and reasonably thorough in their presentation of the facts. To this summary should be added the observation that the nurse has succeeded in effecting a relationship with the patient sufficiently good that, on several occasions, the latter has been able to talk with her about certain aspects of the situation.

A number of questions are raised in any consideration of an episode such as this. How far does the responsibility of the hospital team extend? How far does the responsibility of its individual members? If a rational patient fails to elect the sensible therapeutic procedure that has been recommended, should the matter end there? If it does, should this eventually be considered as a therapeutic failure, just as an unfavorable error in the actual operative technic would be?

In addition to such general questions, two more specific questions arise, having to do with the patient and the nurse, respectively. With regard to the patient, one is led to ask: Is it really accurate to speak of her as "rational" or is this designation an unwarranted assumption? With respect to the nurse, one may ask: What ought her responses to be? That is, what can she say or do, on the various occasions when the patient communicates with her, that will make the greatest possible contribution to the eventual goal—that of gaining the patient's acceptance of operative intervention?

In considering the first of these specific questions, one is faced with a seeming paradox. Under the circumstances, one feels some justification in calling the patient's refusal to give permission to operate irrational. Mrs. C. W. apparently has a clear-cut decision to make, and she chooses the more destructive course. There are marked similarities between such a decision and suicide, which is rarely thought of as a rational act. In this connection, the further point to be noted is that the patient does not even offer the doctors or the nurses anything in the way of a plausible excuse for her decision. Indeed, one is led to suspect that the patient is not herself fully aware of the forces that motivated her decision.

On the other hand, the evidence in favor of considering the patient to be rational is really very strong indeed. Mrs. C. W. is perfectly aware of all that is going on about her. She correctly interprets all that is said to her. She maintains perfectly good, conventional relationships with her family, with hospital personnel, and other patients. Anyone examining her for this purpose would decide very quickly that she is "of sound mind."

One is left, then, with this sort of question: Can a rational person behave in an irrational way? Or, if this question, as stated, is felt to have been clearly answered in the affirmative by the case study, one might ask: *How is it* that a rational person can at times behave in an irrational way? There is also the closely related question alluded to above: Can an individual really be strongly motivated by psychological forces of which he is only partially, or perhaps not at all, aware?

One can see that this line of questioning might have profound implications. It is to the development of answers to such questions, as they have gradually been reached by modern depth psychology, that a number of the following chapters will be devoted.

The questions raised with regard to the responses of the nurse can perhaps be considered more satisfactorily after the balance of the case study has been presented, and the story can be viewed in its entirety.

First, to fill in the material at those points where the numbers were inserted: (1) When the patient asked Miss R. about the exact nature of her disease and the proposed operation, the nurse attempted to read between the lines of the question. If she had not done so, if she had taken the question literally, she would have been prompted by common sense to respond in one of two ways: to have given a direct, factual answer or to have refused to answer and to have referred the patient to the doctor at his next visit. In either case, the response quite likely would have silenced the patient.

However, Nurse R. realized that the patient's real meaning had to be something other than, or at least something more than, the literal one. For one thing, the literal questions as to the nature of the disease and the operation had already been answered by the doctors. For another, technical descriptions of the various possible operative procedures could not in themselves be very meaningful to the patient. What appeared to the nurse as being of much greater significance than the patient's literal questions was her anxiety, the magnitude of which was indicated by her having taken the initiative in seeking the nurse out to talk to at this point. Accordingly, Miss R. did not get bogged down in a lengthy technical discussion; nor, on the other hand, did she adopt a manner in the least hurried or casual. She did not reject the patient by saying that such questions could only be referred to the doctor.

Nurse R. put aside the charting she had been doing and sat down with the patient in an alcove of the ward. She expressed her realization of the tension the doctor's disclosure would naturally produce and her approval of the patient's wanting to talk about the situation. She did respond in a quite brief and simple fashion to the patient's literal questions, but she followed this up with a friendly invitation to the patient to express whatever her troubled thoughts had been. It was at this point that the patient mentioned, among other things, her mother's disturbing terminal illness.

(2) The reference was not fully intelligible to Miss R., since the illness of the patient's mother appeared to be quite different from that of the patient herself. However, Miss R. realized that her own inability to perceive the significance of the patient's reference did not mean that it had none, but rather the reverse, that it had an extremely personal significance and therefore was not immediately intelligible to someone else. The nurse showed an attentive, gently inquiring type of interest at this point, and she refrained from offering the platitudinous type of reassurance that common sense or good intentions might have suggested. In response to this interest, the patient carried her spoken thoughts a step further. She indicated in an indirect fashion that her mother had been incontinent after the stroke, and she reproached herself for not having been as scrupulously thorough in her ministrations to her mother as she ought to have been. At this point her stream of talk came to an end.

Miss R. realized that Mrs. C. W.'s reference to her mother's incontinence could be closely related to her concern over the lesion in her own bowels. She also saw the connection between the patient's helpfulness to others on the ward and her guilty comments about the inadequate care she had given her mother. However, the nurse could not be really sure of the basic significance of what the patient was attempting to communicate. Therefore she was careful not to say too much or to offer a premature opinion about what had been expressed. She did say that she realized that experiences such as those the patient mentioned could make the current situation especially difficult, and she added that she would be available for a chat whenever Mrs. C. W. felt inclined to talk.

(3) In the evening, the patient revealed to the nurse that she had withheld the diagnostic information from her family, and added the comments about her husband and her daughter. Miss R. gained the impression that Mrs. C. W. was somehow more concerned about her daughter than about her husband. The nurse had noticed that the young girl appeared to be somewhat spoiled and perhaps a bit selfish. There seemed to be a close relationship between the patient and her daughter, but somehow the impression had been conveyed that a mixture of feelings, both positive and negative, was involved on both sides. Miss R. thought to herself that the patient might have been trying to spare the daughter in not mentioning the

diagnosis and the planned operation. She also realized that it probably was not coincidence that Mrs. C. W. had revealed concern about *two* mother-daughter relationships that day.

She still felt unsure of all the emotional forces that might be involved in the situation, and of their relative importance, but she took as her cue the apparent identification (i.e., the inner emotional alignment) of the patient with her daughter. Whereas common sense might at this point have suggested that she vigorously urge the patient to break the news to her family and not try to spare the daughter's feelings at such a crisis, Miss R. made a few remarks to the effect that young girls needed a lot of understanding, and then spoke casually for a little while on noncontroversial subjects. By this time the nurse was quite aware that Mrs. C. W.'s disease and the projected operation held a number of very personal deep significances for the patient, in addition to the natural disquiet that such news would hold for anyone.

(4) When reading the surgeon's note in Mrs. C. W.'s chart the following day, Miss R. perceived by its brevity and its tone that the doctors were irritated with the patient and were reacting to her refusal with a sense of its being an unreasonable frustration.

Miss R. and the resident had worked together for over a year, and they held one another in considerable respect. During the conversation in which the resident confided his irritation, the nurse felt free to relate briefly the clues that had been presented to her regarding the patient's emotional conflicts. She mentioned both the distressing significance which Mrs. C. W. attached to the part of her body that was affected and the apprehension which the patient was experiencing in connection with her relationship to her daughter.

The discrepancy between what Mrs. C. W. had offered as the reason for her refusal and the motivations suggested in her conversations with the nurse impressed both Miss R. and the resident. The latter decided that a psychiatric consultation would be the logical procedure under the circumstances now coming to light. The resident asked the nurse if she would inform the patient of this proposal, in view of her having developed such an effective relationship. It was also decided not to press Mrs. C. W. any further for the time being, but to keep her in the hospital for a few days longer.

(5) Accordingly, Miss R. went to speak with Mrs. C. W., who was pretending to read at her bedside. The nurse did not refer directly to the patient's negative decision. She said that the doctors and she could very easily see how upsetting the diagnosis and the treatment recommendations had been to the patient. She added that they were concerned to see her in such distress, and that they had it in mind to ask another one of the hospital doctors (mentioning him by name) to come and talk with Mrs. C. W. She explained that this doctor was especially trained and interested in helping patients whose illnesses presented them with problems too difficult or too upsetting to handle alone. After some initial resistance to the idea, Mrs. C. W. finally accepted it willingly.

The material just presented fills in the gaps at the points where the nurse's responses had been deleted. The events that followed were of equal interest.

Beginning the next day, Mrs. C. W. was seen by the psychiatric consultant. In all, there were six interviews during the ensuing week. During the first several sessions, a number of points originally perceived by Miss R. were confirmed, and some additional material was obtained. It became possible to arrive at an evaluation of the emotional forces involved in Mrs. C. W.'s refusal to give permission for the operation.

It was gradually revealed that the patient had had very mixed feelings toward her own mother, a possessive and demanding woman. Following her stroke, the mother had lingered on as a bedfast invalid for a long time. Mrs. C. W., then in her teens, had had to assume the entire nursing responsibility, and she had done so very conscientiously. The mother was incontinent of urine and feces during much of this period. Although her conscience would not allow her to recognize the fact, Mrs. C. W. experienced intense resentment of the sacrifices demanded of her by her mother. Of these, one that she felt most keenly was having to give up dating during this entire period. Mrs. C. W.'s ministrations to her mother involved almost constant attempts to keep her physically clean.

It became clear to the psychiatrist that Mrs. C. W. had developed severe feelings of guilt over her anger during her mother's trying illness and that these feelings had been intensified at her mother's death. In the current situation—although she had not permitted herself to become fully aware of it—Mrs. C. W. felt that she would occupy her mother's position. Not only would she have to experience a period of invalidism, but also it would be in connection with a disease affecting the bowels. More specifically, in considering the implications of the ileostomy, the patient felt that she would have the same problem (to her, a disgusting one) with regard to incontinence that she had had to face in her mother. Mrs. C. W. feared that her own teenage daughter would feel as she had felt toward her mother. Although Mrs. C. W. was not able to put these thoughts into exact words—was not able, at first, even to perceive them fully—death seemed to be preferable to such an intense reactivation of the old, conflict-laden situation, and a fitting punishment for her having hated her mother.

The mere process of ventilating her feelings and the experience of having an attentive, understanding, and noncondemning listener appeared to be of some value to Mrs. C. W. The first evidence in this direction was that, following the third interview, the patient decided to tell her husband and her daughter about the diagnosis and the treatment recommendations. At this point she still declined to grant operative permission.

In the course of these conversations, the psychiatrist had also inquired about the early relationship between Mrs. C. W. and her mother, that is, about the first years of the patient's life, long before the mother ever had a serious illness. It became clear that even in those years there had been much tension between the two. The mother had been excessively strict and demanding from the very first, although she took the position that everything she did was for the patient's own good. Mrs. C. W. recalled that her mother had been very particular with regard to personal cleanliness. She had been told by her mother with pride that she had been toilet-trained by the time she was ten months of age.

As soon as the patient had taken her family into her confidence, a conference was held, attended by the surgical resident and the intern, the psychiatrist, the head nurse, Miss R., and a hospital social worker. The psychiatrist reported what he had learned and the group began to make plans. The psychiatrist attempted to increase Mrs. C. W.'s awareness of certain of the emotional factors operating in the present crisis which interfered with her making the constructive decision regarding operation. He felt that profound interpretations to the patient about the extent and the first sources of her hostility to her mother would not be acceptable and probably were not required at this point. Nor did the full emotional significance of the fecal incontinence have to be explored. Stress would be placed on the similarity of the two situations in the patient's mind, and on the unrealistic motivations behind the patient's wish to spare her daughter all nursing responsibility. A fuller ventilation of the patient's feeling about her mother and her daughter, and a discussion of the normal relationships between mothers and daughters would be encouraged. A certain degree of reassurance about the naturalness and the harmlessness of the patient's angry feelings toward her mother would be offered.

Since Mrs. C. W. was depressed, it was felt that a certain amount of firmness could also be helpful in the situation, provided that it was untinged by hostility. It was agreed that the surgical resident would supply this quality. After the full discussion of the patient, the resident felt more understanding of Mrs. C. W. and no longer irritated with her. He planned to speak with her in a firm but kind fashion about the shortsighted way in which she had been constrained to regard the situation.

Miss R. took the assignment of helping the patient take a less ominous view of having an ileostomy by seeing that she met several patients in the surgery clinic who had had ileostomies and were doing well, both physically and emotionally.

The social worker agreed to spend some time with the husband and the daughter, particularly the latter, and to help them accept and adjust to the implications of diagnosis, operation, and convalescence. In the event that Mrs. C. W. agreed to the operation, the caseworker undertook to see that a certain amount of practical help would be available on her return home, in the form of arranging daily visits from a visiting nurse. The caseworker explained the existence and the availability of such a resource to Mrs. C. W. at once, in the hope of contributing to the relief of some of the patient's apprehensions.

After an additional several days of effort on the part of the hospital team, Mrs. C. W. accepted the recommendations for surgery. The operation was performed without incident and the patient began a successful convalescence.

Patients with physical illnesses frequently have emotional problems. Those with a primary diagnosis of mental illness may also have a physical condition which needs consideration and attention. It is easy for members of health care professions to focus on the primary illness for which the patient was hospitalized and to be unaware of accompanying conditions. Staff attitudes about mental illness or less serious emotional problems and their acceptance of those suffering with these conditions have a great deal to do with their ability to recognize the patient's afflictions completely. A common misconception is that psychiatry concerns itself only with the management of the mentally ill or those who exhibit behavior which society labels as crazy. Nurses in general hospitals, schools, public health agencies, or industry who believe this are at a disadvantage, for they do not avail themselves of the use of psychiatric concepts in their daily practice of nursing. As a matter of fact, besides caring for and treating the mentally ill, psychiatry is equally concerned with patients in general hospitals who have emotional stresses and problems, and with patients in the community who can be treated without hospitalization. Psychiatry concerns itself not only with the treatment of mental disorders, but also with their cause and prevention. There is a growing emphasis on prevention and early treatment of emotional problems so that more serious forms of breakdown may be averted. Nurses with a good understanding of psychiatric concepts can be most instrumental in assisting with this movement by recognizing and referring for early treatment emotional problems which are yet in their beginning phases.

It is considered poor practice in treating and caring for a patient to neglect considering any aspect of the patient. Nurses must be able to utilize psychiatric concepts in the practice of all facets of nursing so that they may help any patient facing the stress of illness. This is important regardless of whether the primary problem is physical or emotional.

It is sometimes difficult to comprehend why a nurse caring for a physically ill patient is able to show concern and care for him, and at the same time has a great deal of difficulty accepting a patient exhibiting an emotional illness. Such a difference might be explained by looking at cultural norms.

In our culture it is generally more acceptable to have a physical illness than it is to have an emotional one. Yet, both can be equally debilitating and, in fact, in the acute phase, the latter may well have a longer recovery period. Because of this norm, however, one frequently discovers that the physically ill person may have an emotional problem which, because of the stigma against emotional disorders, has been unconsciously translated into a physical manifestation (headaches, backaches, shortness of breath, vomiting, diarrhea, gastric ulcers, acne, to name a few).

It is rarely acceptable for adults to cry or express anger. However, it is acceptable to complain of physical pain or distress which frequently motivates others to come to their aid. The emotionally ill may translate their problems into physical ones which are more acceptable to themselves and others and to which members of the health care professions respond with more sympathy and a willingness to treat.

Nurses who understand basic psychiatric concepts and convey their understanding to the patient will permit the patient to express his feelings more directly. In such an interpersonal climate, patients will find less need to express their feelings through physical symptoms, the attention to which does not relieve the original distress. Nurses and physicians who are unable to accept patients' problems at the emotional, feeling level may well find themselves caught up in the game of "symptom chasing." As one symptom becomes controlled, another, equally distressing, appears to take its place.

All patients are people who, regardless of the type of illness, have the same basic needs to be loved, nurtured, and understood. Nurses who are able to meet these needs will have patients who respond positively to them in their nursing practice.

In many of the nursing specialties, the nurse practitioner is expected to perform technical level functions and procedures for patients which are task-oriented in that they consist of machines and apparatus through which the nurse performs a service for the patient. The measure of professionalism, in these situations, which distinguishes nurses from technicians, is the nurse's ability to move beyond the machine and be primarily concerned about the patient, to recognize and understand the needs of the patient regardless of the level or manner in which these needs express themselves.

One of the most difficult tasks for nursing students and nurses is to understand theoretical, psychiatric concepts in such a way that they might make practical application of these concepts to the nursing situation. The authors will attempt to demonstrate this clearly.

SUMMARY

In her role as a manager, the nurse needs to discover ways to maintain the patient-centered approach and to assist and to encourage other members of the health care team to develop the same philosophy. Because of external and internal pressures, she needs to resist the temptation to give nursing tasks and procedures priority over direct patient care. The nurse needs to maintain or to return to a clinically focused practice which will survive administrative pressures to do otherwise.

Hospitalized patients, whatever the service they may be on, are likely to experience emotional stress as well as physical stress, although nurses and physicians are often insufficiently aware of this fact. Some of the factors that may contribute to the production of the emotional stress include the strangeness of the situation, the draining of energy caused by the physical illness, the loss of self-sufficiency, and the uneasiness aroused by the illness and the prospective treatment. Other contributors to the emotional stress are the alterations in the patient's human relationships, with the loss of habitual sources of support. The outcome of treatment, whatever the nature of the illness, often depends on the ability of nurses and physicians to comprehend the patient as a human being. This ability is by no means wholly intuitive, but requires enhancement through education.

In developing good professional nursing practice, it is imperative that nursing students acquire an appreciation of fundamental, dynamic psychiatric concepts. With this appreciation will come the recognition of the patient's efforts to adjust to the situation at hand. Through understanding some of the basic forces which motivate man to respond or react consciously or unconsciously in a certain manner, the nurse can more clearly comprehend her own feelings and actions and those feelings and actions expressed or demonstrated by others. With this understanding, the nurse should be able to plan for better patient care by being more able to meet the complete needs of the patient rather than by limiting her efforts to one small segment of care. With the understanding of basic psychiatric concepts, the nurse should become more sensitive to the needs of others and have a greater understanding of the conflicts all human beings face in their daily task of living. She may then be able to assist and support patients in their efforts to adapt or adjust effectively.

STUDENT READING SUGGESTIONS

AGUILERA, D. C.: Crisis: Moment of truth. JPN and Ment. Health Serv., 9:23–25, 1971.

CANADAY, M. E.: SSPE—Helping the family cope. Amer. J. Nurs., 72:94–96, 1972.

DAVIS, M. Z.: Socioemotional component of coronary care. Amer. J. Nurs., 72:705–709, 1972.

DETHOMASO, M. T.: Touch power and the screen of loneliness. Persp. in Psych. Care, 9:112–118, 1971.

FRANCIS, H. T.: Leadership experience for ADN students. Amer. J. Nurs., 72:1264–1265, 1972.

FREIBERG, K. H.: How parents react when their child is hospitalized. Amer. J. Nurs., 72:1270–1273, 1972.

GARANT, C.: A basis for care. Amer. J. Nurs., 72:699–701, 1972.

GERMAINE, A.: What makes team nursing tick? J. of Nurs. Adm., 1:46–49 (July-August) 1971.

GOSHEN, C. E.: Your automated future. Amer. J. Nurs., 72:62–67, 1972.

HARDIMAN, M. A.: Interviewing? or social chit-chat? Amer. J. Nurs., 71:1379–1381, 1971.

JOURARD, S. M.: The Transparent Self. Princeton, D. Van Nostrand Co., Inc., 1964.

KOSIK, S. H.: Patient advocacy or fighting the system. Amer. J. Nurs., 72:694–698, 1972.

KRON, T.: Team nursing—how viable is it today? J. of Nurs. Adm., 1:19–22 (November-December) 1971.

KUBLER-ROSS, E.: Dying with dignity. Can. Nurse, 67:31–35 (October) 1971.

LAWLER, J.: "See me, feel me, touch me, heal me." RN, 34:48–49 (September) 1971.

LEVIN, P. and BERNE, E.: Games nurses play. Amer. J. Nurs., 72:483–487, 1972.

LOWENBERG, J. S.: The coping behaviors of fatally ill adolescents and their parents. Nurs. Forum, 9:269–287, 1970.

MAYEROFF, M.: On Caring. New York, Harper & Row, 1972.

MICHAELS, D. R.: Too much in need of support to give any? Amer. J. Nurs., 71:1932–1935, 1971.

MONTAGU, A.: On Being Human. New York, Hawthorn Books, Inc., 1966.

MORRIS, M. and RHODES, M.: Guidelines for the care of confused patients. Amer. J. Nurs., 72: 1630–1633, 1972.

MORRIS, J. and TRABER, W.: After the battle. Amer. J. Nurs., 97–99, 1972.

MURPHY, J. C.: Setting the stage for teaching ancillary personnel. J. of Nurs. Adm., 1:51–54 (November-December) 1971.

MURRAY, RUTH L. E.: Caring. Amer. J. Nurs., 72:1286–1287, 1972.

RAMPHAL, M.: Clinical and administrative judgment. Amer. J. Nurs., 72:1606–1611, 1972.

ROBERTS, H.: Talking to relatives. Nurs. Times, 67:860–861, 1971.

RODGER, B. P.: Therapeutic conversation and posthypnotic suggestion. Amer. J. Nurs., 72:714–717, 1972.

SCHMIDT, J.: Availability: A concept of nursing practice. Amer. J. Nurs., 72:1086–1089, 1972.

SEWARD, E. M.: Preventing postpartum psychosis. Amer. J. Nurs., 72:520–523, 1972.

SHEAHAN, D.: The game of the name: Nurse professional and nurse technician. Nurs. Outlook, 20:440–444, 1972.

SOBEL, D.: Love and pain. Amer. J. Nurs., 72:910–912, 1972.

TITCHENER, J.: Surgery as a Human Experience. New York, Oxford University Press, 1960.

UJHELY, G. B.: Determinants of the Nurse-Patient Relationship. New York, Springer Publishing Co., Inc., 1968.

VELAZQUEZ, J. M.: Alienation. Amer. J. Nurs., 69:301–304, 1969.

VINCENT, P.: Do we want patients to conform? Nurs. Outlook, 18:54–55, 1970.

WHITE, H. C.: Some perceived behavior and attitudes of hospital employees under effective and ineffective supervisors. J. of Nurs. Adm., 1:49–54 (January) 1971.

2

BASIC CONCEPTS OF THE
MIND AND OF MENTAL HEALTH

Adjustment * Mind * Personality *
Behavior * Health * The Mind and Mental Health

The preceding chapter has presented clinical situations that illustrate problems in human behavior. The nurse frequently has the opportunity to play an important part in the solution of these problems. Some practical words of orientation have been given to assist the student in beginning to utilize her relationships with patients in a therapeutic fashion. At a number of points in the presentation thus far, it has probably become apparent that the nurse can obtain the most reliable basis for correct responses when her native intuition and judgment have been reinforced with a sound background in fundamental concepts of the human mind and its workings. This chapter and those that immediately follow are devoted to the development of such a background.

One of the difficulties in presenting the scientific psychology of both the normal and the abnormal lies in the fact that a great many of the technical terms that are indispensable to such a discussion are already in widespread lay usage and therefore have lost the precision of meaning necessary to science. Such terms as *adjustment, mind, personality, behavior, psychology, health, normal,* and *abnormal* fall into this category. It will be helpful at the outset of the discussion to redefine such words, so that they may become the vehicles of useful scientific concepts. Indeed, as is often the case in such matters, a thoughtful attempt to define terms will lead one quite far into the subject matter itself.

ADJUSTMENT

Think for a moment of the never-ending changes to which the human being is called upon to respond if life is to be maintained, pain avoided, comfort sought, and aspirations realized. These changes readily divide themselves into two main groups: changes going on *within* the individual and changes going on all about him, that is, *in his environ-*

ment. From conception until death, the processes of metabolism take place in every cell of the body; the student will have become acquainted with many of these in her courses in physiology and biochemistry. The changes that continuously take place in the environment are no less significant, ranging from such simple physical changes as those in illumination, temperature, and humidity, to the most subtle and complex changes of all, those in human relationships. *The series of technics or processes by which the individual strives to meet these changes and to maintain a satisfactory equilibrium with his world is termed adjustment, or adaptation.*

Notice that changes of either group—the inner or the outer—can affect a "satisfactory equilibrium." Such conditions as hunger and thirst, anxiety and rage, malfunction of an organ or an organ system, can disturb it from within. Excessive heat or cold, infectious agents, the absence of love or the open hostility of others can disturb it from without. Furthermore, as one can readily see from such examples, there is a constant interweaving of inner and outer disturbances, so that the organism is usually called upon to face a combination of problems simultaneously.

If, for example, a camper or explorer finds that an excessively cold environment requires the expenditure of a large part of his time and energy to keep warm, there may be insufficient time and energy remaining to procure food, with the result that hunger arises from within. Similarly, if an individual is faced with a persistent lack of love from the figures in his environment, he may become depressed, with the result that his appetite may be so interfered with that he ceases to eat and becomes malnourished.

Conversely, inner changes can affect one's perceptions of and reactions to environmental changes. A person who is very frightened or angry, for example, may seriously misjudge some aspects of his environment, thereby rendering himself vulnerable to damage from without.

> After a prolonged bout of alcoholic intoxication, a patient was admitted to the hospital in delirium tremens. The patient was toxic and extremely anxious. He misjudged the intentions of an orderly who approached him with an I.V. stand, and jumped through an open window, thinking it was a doorway.

> When fire broke out in a theater, a number of persons became panicky and were trapped, since they were too upset to find the plainly marked exit.

These examples illustrate failures in adjustment, because these individuals were unable to function in a coordinated way. Note that the continuous effort at adjustment requires the organism to function *as a unit*. This type of functioning is termed *mental* or *psychological*.

MIND

In ordinary conversation, *mind* is often used synonymously with brain, or with intelligence, or with consciousness. In scientific usage, one finds that none of these conventional terms is really equivalent to mind, for none is sufficiently inclusive. After all, the brain is a bodily organ; intelligence is a faculty; consciousness is a quality. Mind involves organs, faculties, and qualities of various sorts, but it cannot be synonymous with any one of these.

For example, it is quite true that the central integrative organ of the mind is an anatomic structure, the brain. But the brain is only *one* of the organs of the mind; muscles, tendons, glands, and mucous membranes are also involved. If a person plays tennis, runs for a bus, or answers a question on a quiz program, *all of him* is playing, or running, or answering. In the case of playing tennis (or running for the bus), it is obvious that the action is not merely a function of brain, muscles, or vascular system, but of all of these and more, combined in a single, coordinated effort. Even in such a relatively quiet activity as answering a question, it is clear that the individual is functioning as a total person, one in whom intellectual functioning is combined with vascular and glandular functioning and with the use of the vocal apparatus to produce a unified result.

The example of the quiz contestant also illustrates the error of equating *intelligence* with mind. Regardless of the power of such a faculty, which is rather a complex thing in itself, the individual would be entirely incapable of meeting the situation if he had to rely upon intelligence alone. Without the faculty of perception, the individual could not even become aware of the situation; without emotions, he would not be motivated to meet the situation when perceived; without memory, he could not arrive at an answer to the question, even though motivated to do so.

With regard to the equating of mind with consciousness, there are also insurmountable objections. Chapter 3 will develop this point in detail. However, it can be said here that—as the clinical examples in Chapter 1 revealed—it is possible for an individual's adjustment efforts to be influenced seriously by factors within himself of which he is quite unaware.

Notice that it is virtually impossible to think of mind apart from activity. In other words, mind is a truly *functional* concept. *It is not merely a structure* or a group of structures; nor is it a vague, mystical something apart from the body. It is not a faculty, and it is not a quality, although it may be said to possess faculties and qualities. In plain language, mind is "a person doing something." As a scientific definition, one might say that *mind is a process, complex and continuous; it is no less than the body in action as a unit.*

The terms *mind* and *mental* have been used with a certain looseness even in medical speech and writing. Partly as a result of this carelessness, the expression *mental illness* retains an ominous sound that is usually unwarranted. The image conjured up by the expression is apt to be that of a person who is mad, deranged, perhaps with an organic disease of the brain. To avoid such images, it has become customary to refer to most psychiatric conditions as *emotional illnesses*. This expression is, for the most part, correct enough, inasmuch as emotions are quite centrally involved in nearly all psychiatric disorders. However, as a matter of orientation, it is important for the student using the scientific definition of *mind* to realize that all illnesses in which the patient is affected *as a person,* as a functional unit, are mental illnesses. The term has absolutely no legitimate reference to the severity or the pervasiveness of the disability.

PERSONALITY

In popular usage, *personality* has acquired the meaning of charm or of sexual attractiveness. One says of a popular girl, "She has personality!" Of an unpopular person, one may say, "The trouble with him is, he has no personality." Sometimes the word is used to refer to a combination of likeable or colorful attributes, as when one says, "Susan has a *better* personality than Judy," or, "John has *more* personality than Jim."

In scientific usage, personality has a meaning similar to that of mind but one that is more specific. *Personality refers to the whole group of adjustment technics and equipment that are characteristic for a given individual in meeting the various situations of life.* As will become clearer upon reading subsequent chapters, the words *technics* and *equipment* are used here in a very broad sense and include quite nonmaterial items, such as beliefs, values, and codes of action.

These attributes—technics and equipment—are relatively stable. If one knows a person well, frequently one can predict in a general way, but with considerable accuracy, how he will react in a given situation. On the other hand, personality has a developmental history as well. Over a long period of time, modifications do occur. The personality of an adult is apt to be recognizably similar to that of the same person as a child, but the two are clearly not identical.

It is therefore possible, and in fact necessary, to consider personality from two standpoints. The first is the cross-sectional point of view, in which one attempts to assess the equipment and the technics of adjustment that are currently characteristic of the individual. The other is the longitudinal point of view, in which one attempts to ascertain how the personality came to be what it is. Chapters 3, 4, and 5 will deal primarily with general principles of the personality seen in cross section. Chapters 6 and 7 will be devoted largely to a presentation of personality development. In the study of an individual patient, one uses both points of view.

BEHAVIOR

In any consideration of the processes of adjustment, it is necessary to use the term *behavior.* In everyday speech, the word is used in about the same sense as deportment. Sometimes it is used with the implication of "proper" or "correct" actions, as when one says to a child, "Behave yourself!" or when one speaks of someone as "misbehaving." For the nurse, as for the doctor or the psychologist, it is helpful to define the term more precisely as *all of the activity of a human being that is capable of observation by another person,* or, more simply, as *all motor activity.* Thus it includes obvious and highly coordinated activities, such as those mentioned in the paragraphs on *mind* (playing tennis, running for a bus, and answering a question), as well as such barely noticeable and seemingly isolated activities as a whispered word or the raising of an eyebrow. Although, at first, the significance of any given bit of behavior may be far from clear to the observer, in the final analysis it turns out that most behavior represents a portion of the individual's never-ending attempts at adjustment.

Whereas behavior forms a part of the individual's total adjustment effort, one must remember that this effort includes activities other than those designated as behavior. It obviously includes much *physiologic* activity not directly accessible to the observation of another person as, for example, the secretory activity of the lining of the digestive tract or the changes in diameter of the cerebral blood vessels. It also includes much activity such as ordinary quiet thinking or dreaming, which, though psychological, is not directly accessible to the observation of another and therefore is not behavioral. (However, frequently the subject will present behavioral clues—such as the whispered word or the raised eyebrow—that make it possible for the trained observer to derive some impression as to the nature of the psychological activity that is taking place within. Frequently the subject is also able to make fuller and more deliberate use of such behavioral channels—speech and gestures—in communicating to an observer the nature of his inner psychological activity.)

MENTAL VERSUS PHYSICAL

In a contrasting sense, the use of the terms *physiologic* and *psychological* brings us to a problem that is a legacy of the prescientific era in psychology, the so-called mind-body problem. There has remained a certain amount of confusion and controversy as to which activities of human beings are properly termed *mental* and which *physical*. While the subtler aspects of this question are beyond the scope of this book, it is possible to clarify them sufficiently to aid the student in her thinking and reading.

To begin with, it may be safely stated as a biologic principle that *all* activity of human beings involves physical changes. These changes may be of a very gross nature, such as changes in position of the entire body in running and swimming. They may be of a submicroscopic nature, such as, perhaps, the change in position of a few atoms in a few molecules in cells of the brain when a memory trace is established. A useful way of stating this principle is to say that *all human activity involves physiologic processes and may, at least in theory, be studied from a physiologic point of view.*

Of course, this statement is not to be interpreted as meaning that all human activity is *only* a matter of physiology or that it cannot be studied profitably and interpreted from other points of view, other frameworks of reference. The study of human beings forcibly brings home the truth that "the whole is greater than the sum of its parts." It has been indicated above that whenever the human being is functioning *as such*—that is, as a unit, as a whole organism—the activity in question is properly termed *mental* or *psychological*. It is important to understand that this terminology is perfectly compatible with the recognition that *physiologic* activity of a most complex nature is taking place. Therefore, one may say that *a large part of human activity is mental activity and that it may be studied from both the physiologic and the psychological points of view.*

This psychological frame of reference gives one not merely another way of describing the activity under consideration but, very often, a more effective, more meaningful way than the physiologic. Think for a moment of the example previously given of an individual answering a quiz question, or of any of the following examples: a student working out a problem in algebra; a bridge expert planning the play of a hand; an artist studying a landscape and organizing the composition of a painting. It is almost self-evident that, no matter how advanced the sciences of neurology, biochemistry, and biophysics may become, phenomena such as these can be described more meaningfully in psychological than in physiologic terms.

Perhaps it will have been noticed that, in the examples of psychological activity just cited, the investigator would have to rely for his data almost entirely upon the self-observation and the subsequent communication of the subjects involved. However, in many other examples of psychological activity, such as those mentioned to illustrate the term *behavior*, a large part—perhaps even the most significant part—of what is taking place *is* accessible to direct observation. *Therefore, behavior may be studied from three points of view: the physiologic, the psychological, and the behavioral (that of direct observation).*

HEALTH

Inasmuch as the survival and the well-being of the individual depend on the essential success of his continuous adjustment efforts, on the effective maintenance of a harmonious equilibrium between inner needs and environmental limitations, one can readily arrive at a definition of health in these terms. One may say that *health is successful adjustment and illness represents a failure of adjustment.* The definition is broad enough to include all types of deviation from a state of health, whether these be conventionally labeled mental or physical.

Although such a definition is sound, it is expressed in such general terms as to be of limited practical value. What is needed is to bring it to the everyday clinical level by developing its implications in specific terms. At this point certain difficulties and differences of opinion appear, particularly with regard to the concept of health. Health is always less conspicuous than disease, even as a smoothly running motor is less conspicuous than one badly in need of repairs. The whole problem would be greatly simplified if one could say merely that health is the absence of disease. But as a motor may not be in need of actual repairs and yet may not be running smoothly—needing various delicate adjustments—so a human being may not show clear-cut, obvious symptoms of any kind and yet may not be functioning at his optimum level, may not be enjoying full health.

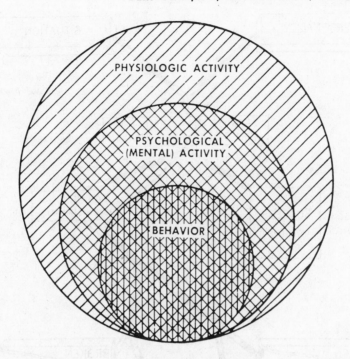

Fig. 2–1. An abstract diagram to illustrate the relationships of various types of activity of the human organism. All activity, whether of the whole or of any of its parts, has a physiologic basis and, theoretically, may be studied from the standpoint of physiology. Thus all activity is shown encompassed within the large circle. Activity of the organism as a whole theoretically may be studied from either or both of two standpoints: physiology and psychology. Activity of this type is shown encompassed by the intermediate circle. A certain portion of psychological activity is accessible to the direct observation of other persons; this activity is termed behavior, and, theoretically, it may be studied from three standpoints: physiologic, psychological, and behavioral. It is shown here encompassed by the smallest circle.

In attempting to simplify the definition of health, one might naturally think of employing a statistical approach. One might define health as the "average" condition of whatever group of human beings one is considering, and illness as an appreciable deviation from this average. For some aspects of the problem this approach works quite well and, in fact, is in general use. For example, if it has been determined that the average red blood cell count among a given part of the population of the United States is 5 million per cubic millimeter, one would be quite correct in attributing disease to an individual found to have a red count of 3 or of 7 million. Similarly, if it has been determined that the average weight of an adult male of a given race is 150 pounds, one would usually be correct in suspecting disease in an individual weighing 100 pounds or in one weighing 250 pounds.

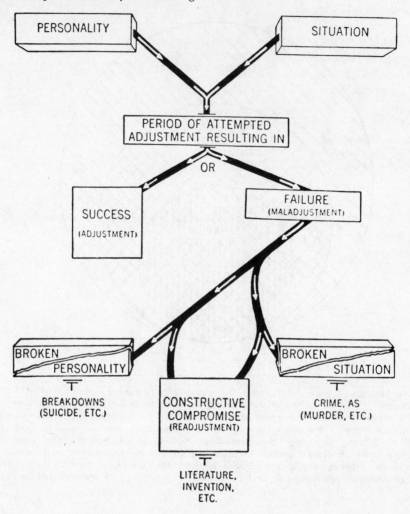

Fig. 2–2. Diagram of adjustment and maladjustment. Health is represented by **success** and by **constructive compromise**. Illness is represented by **broken personality** (psychoneuroses, psychoses, psychosomatic disorders) and, in many cases, by **broken situation** (character and behavior disorders). (Menninger, Karl A.: The Human Mind, ed. 3, p. 31. New York, Knopf, 1945.)

However, if the health student relies entirely on a statistical approach in her definition, she soon encounters serious difficulties. For example, one might do a survey of the red blood cell counts of human beings in certain areas of the world and find entire populations in which the average would be closer to 3 million than to 5 million. It would be a serious error to infer that such a finding in any individual member of such a population represented a healthy condition merely because it was average. In such instances, the health team would quite regularly find that the greater part of the population was suffering from endemic disease, such as malaria, hookworm, malnutrition.

For an example closer to home, one might consider the incidence of infections of the respiratory tract in the population of an industrial city of the Midwest during the winter months. One would probably find that the "average" person would experience two or three such infections each season; in fact, it might easily turn out that a majority of the population at a given time had a mild infection of this type (head cold, sinusitis, sore throat, earache). Yet the error of designating a respiratory infection as healthy on this basis would be obvious. Another example, similar to the above but even more sweeping, is afforded by the incidence of dental caries. Statistical surveys of the oral hygiene of large numbers of adults, such as those conducted in the armed services, reveal that a vast majority of persons have such lesions. Yet, despite such findings, no one would seriously consider dental caries to represent a healthy or a normal condition.

In addition to such instances in which the statistical approach, *used by itself*, breaks down completely, there are other situations in which deviations from the statistical norms signify disease only when they occur in a certain *direction*. In contrast with the matter of the red blood cell count, consider the determination of the intelligence quotient. (This example is the more significant because, intelligence testing represents one of the more successful attempts to apply statistical technics in the field of mental health.) The normal I.Q. of 100 is, of course, an average. One is quite safe in considering an I.Q. of 50 as "unhealthy" (or "abnormal," if the words are used synonymously). But what about an I.Q. of 150?

Mention of intelligence testing leads naturally to consideration of another factor that has an important bearing on the concept of health: *degree of maturity*. As the student will recall from her introductory course in psychology, the most widely used intelligence tests (for example, the Stanford-Binet) have been so developed and standardized that the performance of the individual tested is compared with the performances of other subjects *of the same age*. Thus the numerical value of the I.Q. for any given individual remains a rather fixed quantity, no matter when he is tested. A child of six, let us say, is tested and found to have an I.Q. of 120. The same individual is tested again at age sixteen and still found to have an I.Q. of 120. Yet his intellectual powers *have increased tremendously* during the intervening ten years. Intellectually speaking, his mind *has matured* in the interim. (If such an individual's actual *performance* had been the same at sixteen, as at six, his I.Q. at the latter age would have been not 120, but 38.)

It is the same way with nearly all other aspects of human structure and function. Before arriving at an opinion as to whether or not a given bodily structure or a given bit of behavior represents a state of health, one must take the subject's age into consideration. *That which is quite compatible with health at one age is often a sign of illness at another*.

Another set of factors to be considered in appraising an individual's health has to do with his environment. One cannot form a sound opinion of the effectiveness of adaptive mechanisms unless one understands the factors to which adaptation is required. Again the matter of red blood cell counts furnishes an illustration. Mountaineers typically have red counts far higher than 5 million. This phenomenon is, of course, part of their adaptation to living in an atmosphere with a low oxygen tension. *That which is quite compatible with health under certain circumstances is often a sign of illness under other circumstances.*

It may be helpful at this point to summarize the implications of the material just discussed.

1. It should be clear that *there is no one touchstone or criterion* that the student of human beings may apply to settle the determination of health.

2. It appears that there is usually *no sharp boundary line* between health and disease. As an illustration of this point, one need only refer to the examples of the red count and the intelligence quotient. One feels sure that a red count of 5 million is normal or healthy and that a count of 3 million is abnormal or unhealthy, but what of a count of 4.3 million? One feels sure that an I.Q. of 100 is normal and that one of 50 is abnormal, but what of an I.Q. of 78 or 89.5?

3. When one considers such conditions as head colds, dental caries, and many other minor emotional and physical ailments, one realizes that *absolute health is an ideal,* an abstraction, a goal, rather than something actually achieved. It is much more meaningful to speak of *relative health,* a *relatively* effective adjustment, than it is to attempt to use the term in an absolute sense.

4. In any appraisal of health, one must take into consideration the subject's age and environment.

5. We have found that, although there is no *one* criterion for health, there are several approaches that, *taken together,* begin to offer some basis for evaluation of this question. We can say, for example: (a) that health should exclude established clinical disease entities; (b) that in general it should conform to statistical norms for the population in question (when this point is not in contradiction with the first point); and (c) that it should be based on structure and function appropriate to the age of the individual; that is, it should involve a concept of maturity.

MENTAL HEALTH

Perhaps the student will have noticed that up to this point no attempt has been made to divide the subject of health into mental and physical categories. Such a division is unnecessary and unsound in speaking of general principles, for the principles are the same. However, when one gets down to details, one finds that, insofar as those phenomena of life called mental are more complex than those phenomena directly explainable in physical or chemical terms, the determination of mental health is more complex than the determination of bodily health. *This complexity is especially apparent in two respects: in the evaluation of the effect of environmental influences and in the definition of maturity.*

The problems involved in an evaluation of the effect of environmental influences will receive extended consideration in Chapter 13, but a specific example at this point may be helpful. One rather grave symptom of mental illness is called *delusion*. A simple definition of delusion, frequently encountered in some of the older textbooks, was "a fixed idea, contrary to fact." Such a definition does not take the environment into account. Notice how quickly it breaks down for this very reason. The average European peasant of the fifteenth century had the conviction that the earth was flat. Therefore, could one say that he was deluded and mentally ill? At the present time, primitive peoples in various parts of the world believe that spirits inhabit certain inanimate objects, such as stones, trees, and brooks. Would one be justified in calling such persons ill? In both instances the answer is, of course, a clear-cut No.

On the other hand, if an inhabitant of a metropolitan area of the United States in the twentieth century were seriously to maintain either of these "fixed ideas," one would quite properly begin to have doubts as to his mental health. The factor in the situation that has changed is that of the accepted standards of belief held by the community of which the individual is a member. Although the examples just mentioned are sufficiently striking to permit relatively easy evaluation, the student can readily realize that, in many less obvious instances, the appraisal of environmental, particularly cultural, factors may not be an easy matter.

MENTAL MATURITY

Another aspect in which the determination of mental health is more complex than the determination of bodily health is that of degree of maturity. The student of human behavior is at times envious of the relative ease with which, let us say, the roentgenologist can appraise the degree of maturity of a patient's bony structures. A fuller understanding of the meaning of maturity in mental life must await consideration of the material to be presented in Chapter 6, but at this point certain fundamental ideas can be discussed briefly to illustrate the line of approach.

To begin with, the student would do well to consider those adults of her acquaintance whom she most admires, whose adjustment to life appears to be most successful. Of course, there will be many individual differences among them, but there will also be certain characteristics in common. Among these, the following are apt to be evident: (1) these persons make a realistic appraisal of the situations with which they have to deal; (2) they have effective consciences; (3) they have the ability to love others; (4) they have the ability to find outlets for their own needs. Some enlargement and clarification of these points may be helpful.

1. The close connection between an effective sense of reality and the quality of mental maturity becomes clear when one contrasts adult behavior with that of children. It is quite obvious that children are frequently guided in their appraisal of a situation by their own wishes and fears more than by the environmental (objective) facts. For example, a child's fear of the dark is usually not based on any actual dangers related to the degree of illumination. Similarly, a child's perception of time may be quite unrelated to the objective passage of time when the child is under the influence of a strong wish.

The week preceding Christmas may be subjectively perceived by the child as equivalent to a month at another time of the year.

Of course, the well-adjusted adult has his own wishes and fears, much as the child does, but these wishes and fears do not prevent him from interpreting his environment in terms more closely approximating objective reality. When an adult fails to do this, one can, as a rule, quite readily detect immature—and therefore unhealthy—patterns of adjustment. For example, if a girl carries into adult life a basic fear regarding the attitudes of older women, a doubt of their friendliness and trustworthiness, she may be unable to form an objective appraisal of such women or of their responses to her. A nursing student whose ability to grasp actual situations is influenced by such fears may experience difficulties in her relationships with head nurses and supervisors which are realistically unnecessary. Similarly, a head nurse or a supervisor who has carried into adult life certain fears regarding younger women, having their basis perhaps in an old situation of rivalry with a younger sister, may experience difficulty in arriving at a fair or realistic appraisal of students.

The ability to guide one's behavior by reality rather than by wishes or fears has a number of facets, of which the most significant is the use of long-term rather than short-term values. An individual whose sense of well-being depends to a large extent upon the avoidance of unrealistic fears or the gratification of unrealistic wishes is frequently driven to making decisions that are not in his long-term interest. A woman dominated by the unrealistic fear of adult feminine sexuality may find herself unable to appraise realistically and to respond appropriately to the opportunity for a good marriage. A man dominated by the unrealistic and inordinate wish to please others continually, to have everyone like him, may be unable to respond realistically to opportunities for constructive leadership. In both such instances, decisions may be made that conform to the unrealistic but immediate wishes or fears, but that operate against the best long-range interests of the individual concerned.

2. With regard to the second criterion of mental maturity, that of an effective conscience, it can be said quite simply that the function of a mature conscience is largely preventive; it is to keep the individual out of trouble (not merely in the narrow sense of avoiding punishment, but in the broad sense of preventing behavior that is destructive to himself or others).

A mature conscience is consistent and is able to function on its own in the absence of threats and coercion from the environment. It is not corruptible: it does not take bribes, either from within or without. It discriminates between the current, adult situations and the various childhood situations that the individual has experienced, and it influences the individual along the lines of acceptable adult behavior, even when such behavior would not have been acceptable or perhaps possible for the child.

As an example of an immature conscience, one might consider that of a young woman, who, as a child, was given to understand by her mother that the wearing of makeup was a sign of moral depravity. As a young adult, in a different cultural environment and despite her now believing that there was no sound ethical argument against the use of makeup, the woman found herself almost unable to follow the accepted pattern and wear a certain amount of makeup. When she occasionally forced herself to do so, she felt deeply guilty. In such a case, certainly it could be said that the woman's conscience was *active,* but it could not be said that it was truly *effective,* inasmuch as its dictates did not lead to a good adult adjustment.

It is perhaps worth emphasizing that an effective and mature conscience is not one that never evokes feelings of guilt—far from it. Rather, it is one that evokes feelings of guilt when (a) the feelings are realistic, and (b) the feelings are appropriate *for an adult.* Therefore, it is quite possible in some instances for an effective, mature conscience to evoke feelings of guilt in connection with actions that were *not* associated with such feelings in childhood. As an example, one might consider a young man brought up by his parents to accept without qualms some serious racial prejudices. As a result of sociologic studies in college and favorable experiences with mixed groups in military service, he discards the prejudices. The man's conscience then begins to evoke feelings of guilt in situations that would have been quite comfortable for him as a child; thus it leads him to attempt a constructive modification of such situations.

3. Perhaps the most significant characteristic of the mature personality is its capacity for love. In this context, "love" means all affectionate relationships with other human beings in which their happiness and well-being is taken into account. It is well known that the infant is not capable of love in this sense. The infant has great needs for the affection and the ministrations of others; in other words, he needs *to be loved.* Unfortunately, many adults also have a greater need for love than a capacity to give it; in this particular aspect of mental maturity they have remained infants. Since a person with an inordinate need to be loved frequently endeavors to elicit this response from others in all sorts of ingratiating ways, it may be difficult to distinguish between the need and the capacity.

In connection with the ability to love, it should be mentioned that an adult with this capacity is regularly found to possess a certain degree of liking and acceptance of himself. This does not mean vanity or conceit, but rather a healthy self-esteem, like that implied by Shakespeare in *Hamlet:*

> *This above all: to thine own self be true,*
> *And it must follow, as the night the day,*
> *Thou canst not then be false to any man.*

4. The last major characteristic of the mature personality concerns the fact that all human beings have certain elemental, biologic drives. The sexual drive is one of these; hunger is another; a certain amount of aggressiveness is a third. It is characteristic of the emotionally mature human being that, along with satisfying the other requirements listed above, he will also be able to find appropriate satisfactions for biologic drives. As a result of such outlets, the mature individual functions with relative freedom from distressing inner tensions.

SIGNIFICANCE OF UNDERSTANDING THE BASIC CONCEPTS OF THE MIND AND OF MENTAL HEALTH IN THE NURSING SITUATION

An institutional environment is necessarily different in many ways from a home environment. Such differences can be helpful or distressing to the patient, but there will always be a period of transition and adjustment. To some, a hospital is seen as a refuge, a place of cure, relief, and care, while others may view it as a place of pain or suffering, or a place to die. Regardless of his orientation, the patient will experience the strangeness and the force of the new adjustments called for. The more deeply the patient is concerned about his own condition, the greater his adjustment will be. Consequently, more energy will be required of him physically and emotionally to make the adjustment, so that little may be available to him for relating with his new environment and actively seeking support from it.

It is difficult for the nurse to fully appreciate the degree of stress that hospitalization inflicts upon a patient, because the hospital enviroment poses no particular threat to her. She knows it well, is there of her own choice, and for reasons other than illness. It might be helpful, however, if the nurse would reflect upon her own feelings at the time of her initial exposure to the environment, either as a new student recently separated from home, or as a new or experienced graduate fresh on the job, and try to recall the strangeness and pressures she felt or the difficulties she experienced. This could give her some insight into the dynamics and process of adjustment so that she may understand more clearly the demands this process places upon the patient in addition to the demands of his illness.

The nurse, who is knowledgeable about the requirements for adjustment and the consequences for the individual who experiences difficulty with it, will strive to:

1. _know_ her patients well in order to consciously "assess their equipment and technics of adjustment."

2. _extend_ herself to the patient early in his hospitalization for the purpose of establishing a warm, supportive relationship (with "no strings attached"), that will facilitate his adjustment and sustain him through it. (In other words, the nurse will allow the patient to benefit from her understanding, concern, and care, and not demand that he express gratitude for it or in turn support her.)

3. _anticipate_ his need to understand that which is strange and new to him in his environment and attempt to identify and explore this with him before he needs to "muster up enough courage" to ask. (Many patients, as a matter of pride, are fearful of being perceived by staff as ignorant. They worry or fret for hours over things which concern them rather than make these concerns known for early resolution and resulting, personal ease.)

4. _reassure_ the patient who, because of his condition or illness, is dependent upon others to have his basic needs satisfied. (He needs to know that the head nurse, or members of her staff, will be available to help him when he needs them.)

5. _recognize_ the patient's need to test the staff's commitments to him when he calls

for assistance with apparently insignificant tasks. (This behavior will lessen or disappear as soon as the patient learns to trust staff members and becomes secure in their care. Such trust is facilitated by staff *initiating* the approach to the patient, as a matter of routine, for the purpose of exploring and/or meeting his needs.)

6. _understand_ the significance of the patient's behavior in that it communicates his concerns and feelings to her, while appreciating that there is "more than meets the eye." (Much of a patient's behavior may be studied by direct observation and understood by those astute enough to perceive what is going on with him. However, the physiologic and psychological components of the behavior must also be considered.)

7. _share_ with all members of the health care team her observations and interpretations of the patient's behavior for the purpose of assisting others with their care of the patient as well as securing "consensual validation" in terms of her own professional judgment. (Through consensual validation the nurse is able to view her patients more clearly as they really are. It provides her with a measure by which she can test her views of her patients and subsequently discard her own personal distortions of them. For the most part, these distortions are unconscious and arise from unresolved feelings in the nurse's past.)

It may well be to the student's advantage to review the discussion of this concept which appears earlier in this chapter under the topic of *mental maturity*. Difficulties similar to those described may extend themselves to the patient population. Understanding this phenomenon may more easily explain a nurse's immediate dislike or awe of certain patients. The nurse's realization of this will enable her to approach these patients therapeutically.

8. _validate_ with the patient the inferences she has drawn from her direct observation of him. (This is an essential step in planning for the care of patients. As the patient's history unfolds, it needs to be truly his and not one independently fabricated for him out of the distortions and needs of the health care team.)

9. _plan_ for his care so that what is done for him is uniquely his. (This is possible when the nursing care plan evolves from the nurse's observation of the patient, data she has shared with and gathered from others concerning his condition, and her own needs and knowledge about herself and the possible impact she has on those she ministers to professionally. If ancillary personnel are also responsible for certain aspects of the patient's care, it is important that they be included in the development of the nursing care plan. The nurse should assume responsibility for teaching and directing them, with the same factors under consideration previously discussed, so that the results will be most beneficial for the patient.)

10. _implement_ the plan which includes directing and coordinating the care of other members of the team.

11. _evaluate_ the results of her care and the care of others daily, in an ongoing fashion, so that needed changes in the plan may be considered and brought to the attention of others. (Evaluation of care, in terms of the patient's response to that care, is one of the most essential yet frequently neglected areas in nursing. Possible reasons for this have

been elaborated on in Chapter 1. One could consider changing the title from *Nursing Care Plan* to *Patient Care Plan* which may assist staff members with their task of focusing on patient needs rather than on their own.)

12. *reconstruct* the nursing care plan in areas determined by the evaluation to meet the changing needs of the patient. (If nursing care plans are to be *functional*, they must remain *dynamic*, not *static*. Nurses who do not actively subscribe to this view "the writing of a care plan" as useless paper work required by teachers and supervisors and mandated through hospital policy. The static care plan is truly this, and unless evaluated and changed to meet the needs of patients, may well be better left unwritten.)

The following case illustrates how one nurse attempted to understand the behavior of a newly-admitted patient and began her plan of care to meet the patient's most pressing needs. This involves the use of problem-solving technics, the application of the nurse's knowledge of behavior and feelings, and her ability to listen to and understand what the patient is really saying.

Case 2-1

Mrs. A. B., age 60, was admitted to a two-bed room for treatment of an ulcer on her foot and regulation of her insulin dosage and diet. She had had diabetes for several years, had prided herself that her disease had never interfered with her life and that few of her friends knew that she was diabetic. A widow, she lived alone in her own home, was active in several clubs, traveled a lot, was childless, had a large circle of friends, was a member of the Hospital Auxiliary, and contributed generously to the needs of the hospital.

On admission the only available bed was in a double room; Mrs. A. B.'s roommate, Mrs. D., was a woman of the same age, who was recovering from a mild heart attack. Mrs. D. lived with her school teacher daughter, and supplemented her income by sewing and baby-sitting. Mrs. A. B.'s admission was accomplished with considerable flurry at 3:00 p.m., and the afternoon nurse, Miss P., made her initial visit an hour later and wrote this note.

THE NURSE'S NOTE.   "Mrs. A. B. is very unhappy about her room. Insists that the curtain be drawn between the beds and that a phone be on her table. She has telephoned both her doctor and Mr. S., the administrator, demanding a private room. She has decided to have herself discharged. Refused to allow me to examine her foot because she is not going to stay. Mrs. D. is in tears."

THE NURSE'S INITIAL ACTION.   Miss P. spent some time in the room listening and observing. She allowed Mrs. A. B. to tell her all the things that were wrong, and before leaving she persuaded the patient to stay until after dinner and her doctor's visit. Miss P. spent a little time with Mrs. D., arranged her light for her, and settled her with her newspaper, which she liked to read before dinner. She left the room to study the problem and develop a preliminary plan that would help her clarify her own thinking and assist her in her care of Mrs. A. B. during the next few hours. She drew up her plan, organizing it so that she could add information or modify it as she learned more about the patient.

PROBLEM.   Why was Mrs. A. B. so upset about admission?

Mrs. A. B. Says and Does	Mrs. A. B. May Be Feeling	Nursing Action Indicated
1. "After all that I've done for this place why isn't there a room for me? Please draw the curtain." (Turns on side with back to Mrs. D. and away from nurse)	Neglected Not appreciated Deserted Is unable to extend herself to others at this time	Plan to spend time with Mrs. A. B. to learn ways in which she will feel understood, cared for, and safe. Begin to initiate a warm, supportive relationship.
2. "Why isn't my doctor here? He said he would arrange everything. I don't know why I had to come here. I managed all right so far with **my condition.** I'm not really sick, you know. It's just my foot. I'm too active to stay in bed. How long will I have to be in here?" (Sits up in bed and pushes bedside table away from her)	Lonely Uncertain as to plans and future Angry Has difficulty accepting dependency Appears unable to accept her illness Feels trapped and hemmed in Is accustomed to a wider area of control	Get more information from patient about her illness, how she sees it, what she knows about it, and what she fears. To whom is she directing her anger and how realistic is it? Attempt to state the patient's feelings for her. Needs permission to be dependent when it becomes necessary.
3. "I will be having lots of visitors. I don't want to look like a sick woman with sores. Most of them don't know about **my condition.** What will I say to them? I have always done what the doctor told me." (Pulls bedding up around shoulder)	Is embarrassed by illness Sees illness as an "ugly" thing Feels much less competent Wants her friends to only see her as a well person Feels guilty because of her hospitalization	Does she see illness as a disgrace? Will have to find out early what she does think and know about diabetes. Why does **she** think the ulcer developed? What does she look for in her friends?
4. "Don't send that aide in here again. She wanted to go through my bag. There is not enough space for my things in this little room." (Looks at Mrs. D.'s flowers and cards on the dresser)	Needs to feel in control of herself and her belongings Resents others trespassing on her intended domain Is suspicious of the intentions of others	Will try to help her place her belongings. Needs an explanation about the hospital policy to list all patients' belongings. Discuss in team conference and help the aide learn how to relate more directly with patient concerning her tasks.
5. "Are you the head nurse? Does the Director know I'm here? I'm not used to having just anyone around me?" (Glances in the direction of her roommate, looks at her belongings then looks at the nurse and seems ready to cry)	Very deserted and unappreciated Lonely and afraid and unable to trust people	Must have someone who will stay with her until she can **talk** out some of these feelings and feel better and safer. Communicate to other members of the team what Mrs. A. B. seems to need in a way that will help them accept her and understand her despite what appears to be her haughty attitude. Involve all team members in further developing her care plan. Encourage them to share their observations of her and ideas about her needs with each other.

After Miss P. had completed her preliminary plan, she discussed it with the evening supervisor who had just come to the unit on rounds. In the course of this discussion, Miss P. further elaborated on the situation for the supervisor. It was at this time that several important factors came to light which Miss P. had not yet considered, but which have been alluded to in the description of the case and throughout the recorded dialogue which followed.

The supervisor had questioned Miss P. about the general ward atmosphere at the time of Mrs. A. B.'s admission and asked if she could recall any specific event which may have been particularly distressing to Mrs. A. B. at this time. Miss P. remembered that Mrs. A. B. had arrived on the unit a few minutes before the change of shifts. Therefore, all personnel from Miss P.'s shift, including herself, were receiving the nursing report from the day head nurse so that an aide, about to leave for the day, was assigned to begin the routine admission procedure with the patient. Miss P. confessed that she really did not have a chance to visit the patient immediately following the report because of routine administrative duties which required her attention at the onset of her tour of duty, but "did get to visit her in about an hour." She commented that early in this initial encounter with Mrs. A. B., she was able to identify specific feelings (anger and neglect) in the patient and began to question their focus and cause. During this discussion with the supervisor, Miss P. realized, and was able to state her belief that Mrs. A. B.'s initial feelings of neglect, desertion, and anger could have had much of their origin in her admission experience. This might also explain Mrs. A. B.'s suspicious feelings about the aide which she expressed to Miss P. during their first meeting. Miss P. suspected that the aide was in a hurry to go home and probably rushed through her part of the admission routine (that of listing the patient's valuables and belongings) without an adequate explanation to the patient.

ANALYSIS.   The case under discussion, though stated briefly, is an excellent example of what many patients frequently experience during the course of their admission to a hospital. This is unfortunate, for it contributes to feelings of worthlessness in patients and deters to some degree the early establishment of a therapeutic relationship necessary for their comfort and well-being.

Mrs. A. B. was caught in a system where task- and procedure-oriented staff had placed the accomplishment of such ahead of patient needs. No wonder she felt unwanted and bothersome and that somehow she should have apologized for her very existence on that unit, that day. Staff members communicate these feelings to patients when they place their own needs, or the needs of the hospital, ahead of the needs of those for whose care they are responsible. No wonder Mrs. A. B. felt angry at her physician who had said he would arrange everything. Things did not seem to have been arranged at all, which only added to her feelings of uncertainty as to immediate plans and the future. Then too, as a member of the hospital auxiliary, she had, in the past, contributed generously to the needs of the hospital. Apparently, her efforts had not been appreciated for the hospital did not respond to her in her time of need.

In the discussion on adjustment, the student learned that inner changes can affect one's perceptions of and reactions to environmental changes and that a person who is very frightened or angry may seriously misjudge some aspect of his environment, thereby rendering himself vulnerable to damage from without. Mrs. A. B. was anxious and frightened about her hospitalization. It forced her to look more directly at herself in terms of her disease, and to examine in a more conscious way her own feelings and prejudices about it. Before, she has been able to deny, to a certain extent, the implications of diabetes in relation to the ways the effects of this condition are manifested in the human body. Consequently, the appearance of an ulcer on her foot had been damaging to her own self-image ("I don't want to look like a sick woman with sores."), for Mrs. A. B. had prided herself on the fact that her disease had never interfered with her life.

Many diabetic patients come to believe that society generally views them as having earned the condition with which they are afflicted (the disease is a direct result of something they did wrong, such as overeating as children or adults and becoming obese, or craving sweets and eating large quantities of them without control), that it frequently classifies diabetes with other diseases believed by some to result from "sin" (such as alcoholism, obesity, mental illness, and venereal disease), and that all adverse effects of the disease can be avoided if the diabetic simply follows the physician's orders concerning medication, diet, and routine body care. There is some indication that Mrs. A. B. may have subscribed to this belief for she had only told a few friends that she was diabetic, was concerned about the reactions of those who did not know, should they learn of her condition, appeared to be embarrassed by the illness, and saw it as "ugly."

In view of the theory presented about the process of adjustment, it now becomes clear how Mrs. A. B. could view her admission experience as a personal affront. The poor image she held of herself, because of her beliefs about her illness, had moved to a more conscious level (inner change) and she expected and looked for indications that others held the same view and would, in turn, punish her (affect one's perceptions of and reactions to environmental changes). In other words, she had interpreted the staff members' general insensitivity to the needs of patients and the priority which they assigned to tasks and procedures as a deliberate, malignant act toward her.

Misinterpretations of intended meaning, such as the one just described, lend further support to the philosophy that *patient needs must enjoy the primary focus*. A nurse with a patient centered attitude would have assigned an aide just to talk with Mrs. A. B. in an unhurried manner, until the report was over and she could be relieved by a member of the oncoming shift. This would have helped Mrs. A. B. feel less lonely and deserted and have assisted her with her adjustment to a new and somewhat frightening environment. The relieving staff member, regardless of her training level, would have begun the admission procedure with Mrs. A. B.'s needs foremost in mind. She would have introduced her to her roommate, tactfully helped her establish her territorial rights, offered to help her place her belongings within this territory, and clearly explained to her the hospital's policy of listing all patient's valuables and belongings at the time of admission. During this time, the attending staff member would have listened closely to what Mrs. A. B. was saying in terms of her feelings about herself, her illness, and her hospitalization and would have moved in to reassure her verbally with support and understanding when indicated. Patients need to do more than *talk out* feelings, they also need to know that staff members understand these feelings and to be assured of their interest in meeting the needs expressed by these feelings regardless of the level they present themselves. Such an approach, initially, would have relieved Mrs. A. B. of having to adjust to *needless* environmental pressures. In addition, staff members could have begun a plan of treatment more specifically designed for the presenting physical problem and *its* accompanying emotional components rather than spending time and effort working through a charged situation mostly of their own creation.

THE CONCEPT OF HEALTH APPLIED IN NURSING

In an effort to establish a base from which to measure the degree of health or illness in any individual patient for the purpose of assisting this patient toward optimum health, the student should review the implications listed on p. 28. Note that it is much more meaningful to speak of relative health, or a relatively effective adjustment, than it is to attempt to use either term in an absolute sense, and that, for the sake of evaluation, health can be considered absence of established, clinical disease, conformity to population norms, and behavior appropriate to the age of the individual in question.

As they view their patients, nurses need to be able to differentiate between pathologic, social behavior and the usual life style of each individual. A nurse who is a skillful observer utilizes "wide peripheral vision" (in an abstract sense) in seeking that which is new or unexpected and relates the collected data in ways that might suggest causation. As she formulates plans for therapeutic intervention or care, she should understand and promote attitudes and values conducive to emotional and physical health without imposing her own value system. It is important to realize that if the body is altered through disease, its function is altered. If mind is the totality of function, all disease man has has a mental impact.

Sometimes it is difficult for practitioners of nursing and other allied professions to recognize health and support it as they attempt to eliminate illness. Disease, malfunctions, and maladjustments enjoy a primary focus while the healthy aspects of the mind and body receive little consideration. In fact, there is a real danger that what is considered abnormal in the population at large may well move to the rank of normalcy within the hospital. Members of the health care professions must maintain a constant awareness against communicating to patients expectations of disease-oriented rather than health-oriented behaviors and responses. This is particularly important when dealing with the emotional component of the individual's behavior.

To reinforce health in the individual patient, nurses need to be aware of their own attitudes about what constitutes health and what they consider a healthy response to be. The following case example will lend support to this point of view.

Case 2-2

Mr. O., age 26, has been hospitalized in a large public mental institution since the age of 14. At the time of his admission he was diagnosed schizophrenic and, though limited treatment was offered, he did not respond well. Initially his behavior was erratic and unpredictable and his speech loud, profane, and irrational. In an effort to control (rather than understand) the behavior, large doses of tranquilizers were administered to Mr. O., and he spent many hours in seclusion as treatment of, or punishment for, his assaultive behavior. (There was a standing rule on that unit that all acts of assault, physical or verbal, on the part of a patient resulted in his being secluded regardless of what motivated the assault.)

Over the years, Mr. O.'s behavior gradually changed. He became more manageable (he sat quietly by himself on a bench along the wall and did not react when other patients pushed or bumped against him), and his verbal productions were much less forceful (he spoke very little, but could be heard muttering softly to himself on occasion). His medication had gradually been reduced, and he had not been confined in seclusion for over three years.

Recently a program was introduced to the personnel on Mr. O.'s unit, which emphasized an individual approach to patient care. Mr. O. was seen daily by one of the staff for the purpose of making him feel someone was genuinely interested in him. Within a few months, Mr. O. began to initiate some relevant conversation with other patients and staff and was noticeably more outgoing. He moved about the dayroom at times and began to participate, in a limited way, in some recreational activities on the unit.

On the day in question, Mr. O. was eating on the unit, rather than in the cafeteria, because of an acute upper respiratory infection and fever. He had just begun to eat when Mr. N., another patient who had been quite disturbed for several days, ran up to the table where Mr. O. was seated and proceeded to run his fingers through Mr. O.'s food. Mr. O. reacted with much spontaneity. He jumped to his feet and hit Mr. N., knocking him to the floor, at the same time berating him for his actions, amid much loud profanity and wild gesturing. Several staff members managed to seclude Mr. O., while the nurse phoned for the ward physician, reporting to him that Mr. O. had become quite disturbed, almost like he used to be years ago, that the staff had put him in a seclusion room with some difficulty, where he could be heard swearing loudly and kicking at the door. The physician gave a verbal order for a substantial dose of a tranquilizer to be administered to Mr. O. immediately by intermuscular injection and advised the staff to keep him in seclusion until he settled down.

In analyzing this situation one needs to look at how this staff viewed patient behavior (from what frame of reference) and the ways in which this view was communicated to the patient. In light of staff's treatment of Mr. O. following the mishap, the standing rule concerning patient assault and the nurse's report to the physician and his response, it is apparent that any assaultive behavior on that unit was considered sick and that well behavior was quiet and nonreactive. This was communicated to the patient in the form of a punishment/reward system. Under these circumstances, staff were unable to perceive any health in Mr. O.'s behavior.

As a matter of fact, Mr. O. reacted spontaneously to a situation that most members of the culture would react to should they face a similar experience in their normal daily living. No reaction at all would have been more unhealthy. While it is quite true that Mr. O.'s behavior was more nearly that of a small boy's, one would be pressed to describe what the reaction should be of a normal, 26-year-old male in these circumstances. In our culture, it is considered a mark of manhood to defend one's esteem and physical fighting is considered legitimate and, in fact, encouraged in extreme circumstances.

Mr. O.'s disturbed behavior was *not* like it was years ago, when it was unpredictable and his language profane and irrational. At least in this situation, a response could have been predicted had staff been more aware that Mr. O.'s recent behavior change indicated some healthy growth on his part, and therefore responses to outside pressures would be more likely. With regard to his language, it might have been profane, but at least it *was* directed appropriately toward *real* behavior in a *real* situation.

An unhealthy adjustment to hospitalization spells institutionalization. People with increased dependency, whether physical or emotional, still have or should be encouraged to have a need for maintaining a degree of mastery over their physical and psycho-social environment. As the patient improves, he needs encouragement, support, and help to function in healthier, more mature ways.

In the above situation Mr. O. needed some assurance that his response to the situation had elements of health. He may have needed help in controlling his pentup feelings, for one would not want him to get hurt or to hurt others, but control would come from understanding of and expression of these feelings. Mr. O. had been able to grow thus far because of the love (affectionate relationship) of another human being. This same relationship would have been possible with other staff members if they had approached Mr. O. in a manner that considered his personal well-being.

SUMMARY

Adjustment is defined as the series of processes by which the individual strives to maintain a satisfactory equilibrium in the face of the incessant changes within himself and in his environment.

Mind is the means by which the human organism adjusts; it is the body in action as a unit.

Personality, a term closely related to that of mind, is considered to be the entirety of adjustment technics and equipment that are characteristic of a given individual in meeting the situations of life.

The term behavior is restricted to mean all of the activity of a human being that is capable of observation.

Health is considered to be successful adjustment, and illness to represent a failure of adjustment efforts. There is no single criterion that determines the presence of health. There is no sharp boundary line between health and disease. Absolute health is an ideal, seldom, if ever, achieved. Health should, however, exclude established clinical disease; it should, in general, conform to statistical norms; it should be based upon structure and function appropriate to the age of the individual. Mental health includes all of these criteria. Characteristic of mental maturity are: (1) the ability to appraise reality objectively; (2) possession of an effective conscience; (3) the ability to love others; and (4) the ability to find outlets for basic needs.

Nurses who understand the process of *adjustment* are able to help patients with their adjustment while planning for their individual care. Through an understanding of the concept of *mental maturity*, nurses are more clearly able to analyze their own inter-personal relationships in terms of the way they view supervisors, subordinates and patients, and the impact this view may have on the care of patients. However, as nurses assist patients toward optimum health, they require some knowledge of the concept of health in order to design treatment plans which will support patients to this end.

STUDENT READING SUGGESTIONS

ANDRIOTA, JOSEPH: The development of the concept of mental hygiene. Ment. Hygiene, 39: 657–664, 1955.

BARTHOLOMEW, CLAIRE E.: Preserving your mental and social health. Nurs. World, 132:25–26, 1958.

BERLIEN, IVAN C.: Growth as related to mental health. Amer. J. Nurs., 56:1142–1145, 1956.

DENNIS, LORRAINE: Psychology of Human Behavior for Nurses. Philadelphia, W. B. Saunders, 1962.

GRIFFIN, J. D.: Mental health and its changing perspectives. Can. Ment. Health, 19:3–7, 1971.

GUBRIUM, J. F.: Self-conceptions of mental health among the aged. Ment. Hygiene, 55:398–403, 1971.

HAGERMAN, Z.: The concept of love as it relates to nursing intervention, pp. 61–71. In Zerad, L. and Belcher, H. C.: Developing Behavioral Concepts in Nursing. Atlanta, Southern Regional Education Board, 1968.

HAUN, PAUL: Mental health for living. Nurs. Outlook, 5:512–515, 1957.

MASLOW, A. H. AND MITTELMANN, B.: Principles of Abnormal Psychology, rev. ed., pp. 12–21. New York, Harper & Row, 1951.

MENNINGER, K. A.: The Human Mind, pp. 21–34. New York, Knopf, 1945.

NUTTIN, JOSEPH: Psychoanalysis and Personality, pp. 205–232. New York, Sheed and Ward, 1953.

OFFER, D. AND SABSHIN, M.: Normality: Theoretical and Clinical Concepts of Mental Health. New York, Basic Books Inc., 1966.

SAUL, LEON: Bases of Human Behavior, pp. 99–104. Philadelphia, J. B. Lippincott, 1951.

SCHMIDT, M. D.: How industry can promote good mental health—a nurse's viewpoint. Occup. Health Nurs., 19:12–14 (July) 1971.

SIEGEL, H.: The universe of health: A conceptualization. Nurs. Forum., 10:32–35, 1971.

VONACHEN, HAROLD A. AND MASON, JOSEPH M.: The employee's mental health. Amer. J. Nurs., 57:758–759, 1957.

3

FUNDAMENTAL DYNAMIC CONCEPTS:
LEVELS OF AWARENESS

It is our less conscious thought and our less conscious actions which mainly mould our lives and the lives of those who spring from us.

—SAMUEL BUTLER*

Unconscious Mental Activity * Repression

Perhaps the most fundamental characteristic of modern psychology, psychiatry, and psychiatrically-oriented medicine and nursing is the one designated by the term *dynamic*. Professionals in the field of human behavior today are no longer content merely to describe and catalogue the varieties of activities and experiences that comprise human life. It is felt that now one can and should go further than this: one can and should go on to an understanding of the *forces* that move human beings to the activities and the experiences. The term dynamic is used to indicate this interest in the nature and the operation of the driving forces. As will be shown in the present chapter, these forces frequently operate without the subject's awareness of them; hence, for example, a *dynamic psychiatry* or *psychology* has come to mean one that takes into account the importance of unconscious forces within the personality.

In Chapter 1, during the discussion of Mrs. C. W., the patient with carcinoma of the bowel, the question was first raised as to whether or not a person could act on the basis of motivations of which he was unaware. The concept of levels of awareness in mental life is one so fundamental to modern psychology as to warrant careful consideration. Three levels, or degrees, of awareness are involved, and are called: *conscious, preconscious,* and *unconscious.*† By conscious is meant all mental activity (thoughts, sensations, emotions)

---

* *The Way of All Flesh.* New York, Doubleday.

† The term subconscious, which somehow has made its way into popular usage, has no clear scientific meaning and should be avoided.

of which one is aware or can become aware with little or no effort. By preconscious is meant all mental activity of which one is not aware but which can be brought into awareness with effort. Preconscious material is referred to when one says: "It's on the tip of my tongue," or "I know that I know it, but I just can't say it at the moment." By unconscious is meant all the rest—by far the largest fraction—of mental activity or mental life. Unconscious material is registered somewhere in the mind but cannot be brought into awareness by any direct effort, no matter how vigorous.

UNCONSCIOUS MENTAL ACTIVITY

For a long time certain intuitively gifted men—poets, artists, philosophers, prophets— have implied or even expressed the belief that important aspects of mental life could exist below the threshold of consciousness. This idea can be quite disconcerting, however, and it has gained a secure place in the field of science only within the past 60 years or so. For a long time mental and conscious were generally regarded and treated as synonyms, and it is not difficult to see why this should have been the case. There have been two sorts of reasons to account for the long delay on the part of science in recognizing the existence and the power of mental forces below the threshold of awareness. The first was simply the lack of technics for demonstrating such forces. The situation here was quite comparable with that in other branches of biology and its applied specialties, medicine and nursing. As an example, consider for a moment the development of knowledge about muscle function. Even primitive man had a considerable amount of information about the gross functioning of the muscles of his body: he knew a lot about factors influencing speed, endurance, coordination, and so on. As soon as gross dissection of bodies was practiced, as, for example, in certain Greek schools of medicine, much more information was added. However, it was not until quite recently that the really significant finer points about muscle structure and function have been understood. The structure of the individual muscle cell could not be perceived until the development and the application of the microscope. The essentials of muscle metabolism could not be ascertained until the development of the highly refined technics of modern biochemistry. It has been only within the past 60 years that psychological technics of observation and analysis have been developed which are comparable with the anatomist's microscope and the biochemist's microtechnics.

But a second factor, much more significant than the purely technical difficulties, has steadily interfered with the acceptance and the utilization of the concept of unconscious mental processes. This is the need for personal security and comfort. Most of us find it interesting to learn about our bodies. As a rule, we are not made uneasy by the recognition that there is a lot more to learn about the ways in which our muscles, glands, and other organs function than we at first suspected. But it is somehow rather different closer to home so to speak, when we begin to study the mind. Most of us like to feel that we "know our own minds," that is, "know ourselves," quite well. We can accept the fact that life is full of surprises, but we prefer to have the surprises come from outside ourselves, not from within.

When one first hears the suggestion that much of one's own mental functioning goes on without one's being aware of it, one may experience an entirely natural wish to disbelieve. It is this wish not to believe that has constituted the second sort of difficulty. Until the uneasy feelings giving rise to the wish can be dispelled, the wish not to believe persists and can prevent any useful understanding of the levels-of-awareness concept. This circumstance accounts for the fact that many doctors and nurses have an intellectual grasp of the concept and can even use it rather glibly in talking about patients or themselves, without really being able to put the concept to work for them in practice. Fortunately, there are good answers to the problem created by the uneasy feelings, but these answers are perhaps better postponed until the evidence regarding the validity of the levels-of-awareness concept has been presented.

A good starting point in the consideration of such evidence is to be found in certain minor "errors" of everyday life. Here are some examples from real life:

A harried businessman labors under the impression that a woman's lot in general, and that of his wife in particular, is a good bit easier than his own. One morning in December his wife hands him a batch of Christmas cards with instructions to mail them without delay. Thinking of his busy day's schedule, he momentarily regards the chore as an imposition, but he realizes that the cards should be sent and promptly agrees to post them. . . . Some weeks later, when taking his overcoat to the cleaner's, he discovers the cards in an inside pocket.

A college boy, serious about his work but somewhat behind in his studies at the moment, considers how he will spend a weekday evening: calling on his girl friend or going to the library to study. He decides that, everything considered, the latter is much the wiser course. He gets in the family car, drives a few blocks absentmindedly . . . and finds that he has pulled up in front of the girl's house.

A student nurse, at a school whose dean was considered an unpleasant tyrant, had the misfortune (?) to park her car in the space reserved for the dean's use. She returned to find on the windshield a sharply worded note from the dean, advising her to be more careful in the future. Although she disliked the dean, this feeling seemed to be quite outweighed by the fear that she might have jeopardized her school standing, and the student decided to call up and apologize. . . . Only after she had hung up did the girl realize that she had said, "Dean ————, I'm terribly sorry that I parked in your *plot* this afternoon!"

On arising and seeing that it was a beautiful day, a doctor was fleetingly aware of the wish to spend the morning on the golf links instead of making hospital calls. From long habit he promptly forgot the impulse and, as he started for the garage after breakfast, he was conscious only of a mild impatience to get started with his day's work. . . . Yet he found that he had carelessly left his car keys on the bureau. When he had retrieved the keys and was starting the car, he realized that he had mislaid his appointment book.

Slips and errors of the sort just described are extremely commonplace: all of us have occasionally done something similar. They are usually amusing to everyone except the person making the error. As a matter of fact, comedians have used this principle for a long time as a laughter-getting device. Now what are the essential elements of this type of behavior? Think of the four examples: a man forgets to mail some cards; a boy shows up at his girl's house; a student tells a disliked authority figure that she has a "plot" (cemetary lot); a doctor is delayed in getting to work. In each instance there is strong evidence to suggest that the resulting action is in accord with a wish of the person involved. In each instance the subject is unaware of any such intention *at the time the action occurs.* The harried businessman would have said that he had every intention of mailing the Christmas cards, that, everything considered, he "wanted" to mail them. The young student would have said that he "meant" to drive to the library. The student nurse would have said that she wanted to apologize to the dean, not to express dislike of her and certainly not to wish her dead. The doctor would have said that he had given up the idea of playing golf without a moment's hesitation and was actually eager to get to work.

Since the wish, in all four of these instances, was not in the subject's awareness at the time it governed his behavior, it cannot be considered conscious. However, since the wish could subsequently be recalled (with varying degrees of effort), it cannot have been truly unconscious. Therefore, the wish belongs in that border zone called preconscious.

As the last example shows, professional persons are by no means immune to such experiences. A little thought will probably recall to every student a number of medical and nursing errors that clearly fall into this category. Here are a few illustrations:

A resident has had considerable difficulty with a certain patient who is ill-tempered, querulous, and constantly complaining of pain and lack of attention. It is the resident's belief that the patient is not actually in pain but is merely using this complaint as a technic of enforcing his numerous requests. A staff physician, having examined the patient, comes to the conclusion that the pain is caused by a real physical lesion. He explains the basis for his belief to the resident and instructs the latter to write a p.r.n. order for aspirin and codeine. The resident respects the staff man's judgment, accepts the recommendation, and believes that he has mastered his irritation with the patient. A day later, when the order book is reviewed, it is noticed that the p.r.n. order has been written for aspirin alone.

A doctor is consulted by an old and admired friend with whom he has been on very close terms. The friend complains of a chronic cough. He is known to be somewhat allergic and to be a heavy smoker. The doctor examines his friend, has him cut down his smoking, and treats the allergy. The cough persists. The doctor suddenly realizes that he has neglected to have a chest roentgenogram made. When this procedure is done, the presence of lung cancer is revealed. In reviewing the case at this point, the doctor comes to the painful recognition that his uncharacteristic omission of the roentgenologic examination at the first consultation was based on dread of what might be found. The doctor himself is a heavy smoker.

A nurse, working on a convalescent ward, is attracted to the resident and enjoys the opportunity of working with him. One day she finds to her disappointment that her hours have been changed to the 11:00 P.M. to 7:00 A.M. shift, a change that eliminates this opportunity. On taking off her uniform after the rest period on night duty, the nurse finds that she has walked off with the narcotic keys in her pocket and therefore has a reason for returning to the ward in the daytime.

A point worth noting in all seven of these examples is the *nature* of the wish, the impulse, or the tendency that has remained below the threshold of awareness. Think again of what was involved in the various illustrations: irritation with one's wife; being with the girl friend in preference to doing needed study; anger at the dean; the wish to play in preference to the wish to work; resentment of a patient; the dread of discovering serious or fatal illness in a dear friend, plus the dread of developing such an illness one-self; romantic interest in preference to good nursing procedure. It is all very human, but notice that in all instances the material kept out of awareness is, either in itself or under the existing circumstances, disturbing. It is against one's conscience, or against one's best (long-term) interest, or it is directly productive of anxiety. The implication is clear: experiences such as these do not represent the workings of blind chance. Not only is the material that is put or kept out of awareness meaningful, but its *being* put or kept out of awareness is also meaningful. There is a shorter and more scientific expression for the cumbersome phrase "put or kept out of awareness." It is *repression.*

A deed knocks first at thought,
And then it knocks at will.
That is the manufacturing spot,
And will at home and well.

It then goes out an act,
Or is entombed so still
That only to the ear of God
Its doom is audible.
—Emily Dickinson

REPRESSION

It is important to realize that the act of repression occurs automatically, not voluntarily. The truth of this statement is perhaps most easily discernible in the sixth example given above. There can be no question that the doctor's conscious intention, from first to last, was to use the wisest and most scientific approach to his friend's illness. There was no conscious thought whatever of excluding alarming possibilities from consideration. The doctor had no intention of protecting his own sensibilities by ignoring his friend's disease. The automatic, involuntary nature of repression can also be demonstrated in the other examples; perhaps a consideration of the first will suffice to make the point clear. The harried businessman was momentarily aware of irritation with his wife, but he did not stop to explore this feeling, to see how strong it was or how deep it went. Nor did he make the resolve to put the angry feeling out of his mind or to be on guard for any betrayal of it in his actions. He was aware only of having made the simple, almost instantaneous decision to mail the cards because it was the only logical thing to do.

Perhaps the reader has noticed that the example of the doctor and his friend with the chronic cough, unlike the other examples, affords considerable room for doubt that the hidden feeling influencing the doctor's behavior had come to the surface even transiently during the first consultation. Further, the experiences that caused the doctor to become aware of his hidden motivations—namely, the persistence of his friend's illness and finally the grim x-ray picture—were of an exceptionally jarring nature, much more so than in any of the other examples. There is thus the real possibility that this particular illustration involves material that was not merely preconscious but actually unconscious.

A series of analogous examples could be presented to illustrate behavior primarily or entirely motivated by wishes or fears in that deeper layer below the threshold of awareness designated as unconscious. In such a series of examples, the subjects would be quite unable, unless assisted by psychotherapy or by some startling or unusual combination of circumstances, to arrive at an understanding of the behavior in question. The following illustration is typical of such a series:

> A young doctor, in generally good emotional and physical health had noticed and, on occasion, remarked to his friends, that all of his life he had felt an automatic, "instinctive" dislike of older men with certain physical characteristics: a swarthy complexion and dark body hair. In several individual cases in which he got to know such a person better, he was able to assure himself that no objective grounds whatever existed to account for his unfavorable and unpleasant emotional reaction. Even here, the feeling did not entirely disappear, and knowledge of it was a source of embarrassment.
>
> At a later period, in connection with his psychiatric training, the doctor underwent a personal psychoanalysis. This experience involved the release of many long-forgotten memories, one of which threw light on the unwanted reaction just described. The doctor recalled that, at the age of four years, during a family crisis, he had spent several days in the home of a cousin of his father's, a man with a swarthy complexion and dark hair, who had treated him in a cruel and frightening fashion. The doctor had not seen this man in twenty years and for most of this time had completely forgotten the disturbing episode.
>
> Although the young doctor continued to feel that the older man's treatment of him as a small boy had been wrong, he found that his automatic dislike of persons with similar bodily characteristics came to an end.

In this example one notes that the mental material—an unhappy and frightening memory that influenced the subject's responses in a way that was against his intentions and against his best interests—remained entirely below the threshold of awareness for a long period of time. Further, it remained so buried, despite the subject's having given a certain amount of thought to the problem it created, and despite his having tried to figure it out.

Another line of evidence to be considered with regard to the question of levels of awareness does not come from everyday behavior nor from treatment records, but from certain types of psychological experiments: conditioned reflexes and hypnosis.

As most readers will recall, conditioned-reflex experiments can be performed with either animal or human subjects and can be of a very simple nature. If, as in the classic example, a dog is repeatedly offered food at the same time that a buzzer is sounded, after a certain number of feedings salivation can be produced by the sound of the buzzer alone. Exactly the same experiment can be performed with a hungry human subject, and the result will be the same. Of course, the sight and the smell of the food, the sound of the buzzer, and the salivation would all be quite conscious. But now consider the following experiment. The human eye exhibits a pupillary reflex in connection with the amount of illumination present, contracting in bright light and expanding in darkness. A subject can be placed in an experimental situation in which pupillary contraction is repeatedly produced by an artificial light while, at the same time, another stimulus of minimum intensity, let us say a very faint scratching noise, is offered. The latter stimulus can be so weak as to be absolutely below the subject's threshold of awareness. The proper gradation of such a stimulus—loud enough to be registered somewhere in the mind and yet soft enough not to arouse the subject's attention—is not a difficult matter, as can readily be realized when one considers the thousand and one sights, sounds, and smells in one's environment all the time that are not attended to.

After this combination of the bright light and the very faint sound has been presented simultaneously to the subject many times, pupillary contraction can be produced in the subject by the very faint sound alone. This effect can be achieved without the subjects having been aware of the conditioning and without his being aware of the conditioned response when it is produced.

Here, one has an example of mental activity—on a very simple level, of course—that takes place in an entirely unconscious fashion. (In this instance *repression* plays no part, since there is nothing to be "put or kept out of awareness"; there is no conflict of motivations.)

Although the following experiment is in itself simple, hypnosis affords good evidence that a much more complex type of mental activity than an optical reflex can exist far below the threshold of awareness.

A subject is placed in a deep hypnotic trance. Then he is instructed by the hypnotist that, five minutes after awakening, he will be seized by an inordinate thirst and will ask for a glass of water. He is further instructed that he will be completely unable to recall his experiences during the trance until after he has drunk the water. Then the subject is awakened.

During the next few minutes he is questioned about his bodily sensations such as thirst and reports nothing at all unusual. He is asked to report what occurred during the trance and cannot do so. After approximately five minutes, the subject says that he has suddenly become very thirsty and must have a glass of water. After drinking the water, he recalls the entire experience.

Hypnosis is an area of considerable interest, both practical (therapeutic) and theoretic, and an experiment such as the one just cited can raise a whole series of questions. However, for the present purpose, it is important to focus on a single aspect of the situation. An idea, that of intense thirst, was given to the subject. At the moment the idea was offered by the hypnotist, the subject was quite aware of it: he (consciously) understood it. Five minutes after awakening, the subject was strongly affected by the idea and the sensation that it produced. But between the moment of awakening and the end of the five-minute period, the subject was not aware, and was unable by any amount of effort of his own to become aware, of the idea that he would suddenly become thirsty and ask for a glass of water. In evaluating experiments of this type, the inference that *an idea can be completely unconscious and yet be completely effective in determining an individual's behavior* is inescapable. (In this instance the hypnotist's statement that the subject will be unable to recall the trance experiences for a period of time may be regarded as having artificially induced repression.)

The conditioning and the hypnosis experiments bring to mind a controversy that has received much publicity and that involves psychological activity of which the subject is unaware: subliminal advertising. Trials have been made through the television and radio media in which advertising suggestions were presented, using visual or auditory stimuli, frequently repeated but too weak to be consciously perceived by the audience, during the course of an ordinary program. It was found that many members of the audience were in some measure influenced by the subliminal suggestions.

There is, then, very sound evidence for believing that phenomena of mental life can take place in any of three strata with regard to the attribute of awareness: conscious, preconscious, and unconscious. This subject will be explored further and utilized frequently in the chapters to follow, but it is appropriate to consider two additional aspects at this point. The first is the variety and the richness of the material that may exist at preconscious and unconscious levels. Even from the relatively few examples presented in this chapter, one can obtain some notion on this score. Certainly, emotions can be present: irritation and anger, romantic or sexual feelings, and anxiety were all in evidence. Ideational material can also be present. As a matter of fact, all those varieties of mental life that one has been accustomed to associate with consciousness can exist preconsciously or unconsciously; and, as mentioned earlier, the actual amount of mental activity that goes on below the threshold of awareness is far greater than that of which the individual is directly conscious. To illustrate this point, sometimes the picturesque analogy has been made between the mind and an iceberg, in which the conscious mind is likened to that portion of the iceberg that is exposed to view above the level of the sea, and the unconscious to that far larger portion of the iceberg that remains hidden from view.

A second point that may be helpful at this stage concerns the interrelationship of the three strata. Before this can be discussed, a few comments about terms are in order. Although it is convenient to use such terms as *levels* or *strata,* it should be stressed that such usage is really only a figure of speech, much like the iceberg analogy. When one speaks of mental activity as being conscious, preconscious, or unconscious, one is not referring to *structure* in any sense. No anatomic reference is implied. Furthermore, no concept of structure, even in a theoretic sense, is as yet involved. Theoretic concepts of the "structure of the mind" do exist. At times they can be quite helpful, and material of this sort will be presented in Chapter 5. It is, however, important to remember that the terms conscious, preconscious, and unconscious serve merely to describe an *attribute* of the bit of mental material in question.

This attribute is subject to change. A given thought, a feeling, or a wish may at one point in an individual's life have the quality of being in consciousness. At another time, under different circumstances, it may be preconscious, or it may be unconscious. The examples given in this chapter illustrate this changeability of a given bit of material with respect to the degree of the subject's awareness. In the examples having to do with errors of everyday life, certain wishes or feelings were at first (for the most part) quite conscious in the minds of the individuals concerned. They then dropped into the preconscious layer. While preconscious, they exerted an undesired influence on the individual's behavior. The unexpected behavior stimulated the subject into a realization of the preconscious wish or feeling. That is, the shock of the unexpected behavior produced *insight* on the individual's part into what his motivation had just been: the motivation again became conscious.

Similarly, in the case of the hypnotized subject, an idea—that he would become thirsty and ask for water—was at first conscious, then completely unconscious, and again conscious.

There is reason to believe that in every human being a continuous process of shifting or interchange of material between the three layers takes place. As indicated above, the individual's voluntary efforts are only very partially responsible for effecting such shifts. Nor are the shifts in levels of awareness the result of chance. Rather, such changes are the result of a combination of forces, some internal and some external. The exact nature of these various elements will be discussed in future chapters.

The reader will recall that earlier in this chapter reference was made to two factors that have served to hinder the development and the recognition of the levels-of-awareness concept. The first, or technical, factor has been eliminated. The second is personal, the naive but sincere wish not to believe, based on anxiety at the idea that one may be unaware of the motivational forces working within him. On the basis of the previous material, it is now possible to offer considerations to offset the second factor.

These considerations fall under two heads: the value of the levels-of-awareness concept in understanding and helping others, and the value of the concept in understanding oneself and thus establishing a more secure position from which to take action.

Very likely it can already be seen how far-reaching are the implications of the concept in the understanding of patients and in the interpersonal relationships that play such a decisive role in the profession of nursing. The realization that an individual may at times be quite unaware of the real motivations for certain features of his behavior may be of great value to the nurse. Quite often, for example, what a patient may offer as the reason for a given response may be very largely a rationalization. Indeed, the actual motivations for a considerable amount of behavior that strikes one as unreasonable are unconscious. As a case in point, very likely it can now be accepted that the forces influencing Mrs. C. W., the patient with bowel cancer, were largely unconscious. It can be seen that this was one of the premises on which Nurse R.'s successful management of the situation depended.

The advantages to the nurse of this realization of the power of unconscious forces are quite profound. Since it is clear that a person cannot bring his powers of conscious logic to bear on motivations that are largely or entirely unconscious, it is very apt to be a waste of time to become argumentative or to try to "reason it out" with a patient acting under the influence of such motivations. Moreover, such a procedure is frustrating and irritating to the nurse or the doctor as well as to the patient, and this frustration and irritation can be largely avoided.

In addition, the possibilities for a truer and more meaningful understanding of the patient are greatly enhanced. One finds it worthwhile to do a good bit of relaxed listening and to be on the alert for clues as to the unconscious and the preconscious forces at work in the patient. In a sense, everyone retains the wish to be understood, even in many of those aspects of his behavior that are not completely clear to himself. The more the nurse can convey of acceptance and a wish to understand, the more the patient will reveal of himself. The knowledge that motivational forces below the threshold of the patient's awareness can be influencing his behavior adds a new dimension to the nurse's skill. It will be a rewarding surprise to the nurse to see how many times this knowledge will spare her the occasion of having her feelings wounded or her temper aroused. Frequently, it will allow her to feel relaxed and unthreatened in situations that otherwise would have been taken as personally offensive.

Although it is, on the whole, considerably easier to cultivate an awareness of unconscious forces in the behavior of others than in *one's own* behavior, the latter is also possible, and it pays large dividends in the form of increased effectiveness. It paves the way for an assessment of one's own reaction patterns, making possible a type of learning and professional advancement not to be obtained otherwise. Understanding some of the deeper aspects of one's own personality permits one to be far more helpful to patients— through being able to make allowances for one's own imperfections—than would otherwise be possible.

. . . first cast out the beam out of thine own eye and then shalt thou see clearly to cast out the mote out of thy brother's eye.

—MATTHEW, 7:5

It has been said that knowledge is power. The achievements that self-knowledge makes possible form a most significant example of the truth of this statement. Once one has become convinced of the existence of unconscious motivational forces, the cultivation of an awareness of these forces in oneself eventually produces an ease and a security that the ignoring of them can never attain. This promise constitutes the best answer to the initial skepticism, born of anxiety, that makes everyone inclined resist the levels-of-awareness concept.

The following case illustrates situations which many nurses or nursing students have experienced to some extent during their training or professional careers and is an attempt to elaborate descriptively on some of the foregoing theory.

Case 3-1

For several years Miss J. had been head nurse of the surgical ward in a large city hospital and was generally considered by the nursing office and attending physician staff to be competent. She seemed to be efficient in organizing her unit in that routine admissions and emergencies appeared to be accommodated with considerable ease, patients returning from surgery "slid into their proper slots" with little apparent trouble, and nursing tasks and procedures were completed at the end of her shift.

The unit supervisor, Miss K., an elderly woman of 25 years of service, whose retirement was a few months away viewed Miss J. as somewhat of a godsend. It is true that Miss K. had heard vague reports suggesting, that at times, Miss J. exhibited a brisk, unfeeling attitude toward patients and their families, "but," thought Miss K., "she was much better than her predecessor who flew about at loose ends, always needing additional help and rarely getting her duties completed at all. At least Miss J. was not constantly demanding supervisory support and assistance when there were so many other units to attend to. Anyway, in light of her efficiency, how could Miss J. be constantly concerned with and aware of patient's feelings? Emphasizing one would naturally cause some sacrifice with the other." (Miss K., in her role of supervisor, saw herself more as an on-the-spot trouble shooter than as one who worked at helping staff eliminate the source of the problem.) She approached problems in terms of their symptoms, and, consequently, only dealt with what presented itself in the "here and now." She had little knowledge or understanding of human behavior and therefore was unable to assess or assist her staff with assessing any situation in terms of this component.

Miss J. liked her supervisor because Miss K. left her pretty much alone. Miss J. enjoyed this kind of independence, for in the past she had had trouble with authority figures, particularly when they became too directive or controlling and questioned her about her care of patients. Miss J. felt that she was a good nurse and reacted to most supervision from her superiors with righteous indignation. She generally viewed them as spies, waiting for her to do something wrong so they could bring it to her attention and reprimand her for it. (Once, she inadvertently referred to one of her supervisors as "the snoopervisor" when she asked the telephone operator to page her for an emergency. She realized immediately what she had done and was both surprised and embarrassed. The operator's giggle, indicating that she had understood what she said, only added to her discomfort, for Miss J. could not be sure the operator would not tell the supervisor, and if she did, Miss J. felt she would be in trouble. She had forgotten, until that incident, that as students, she and her friends frequently referred, among themselves, to those with authority as "snoopervisors." Miss J. was quite dismayed for she could not be sure she would not slip again.)

Miss J. was uncertain why she reacted or felt as she did when some people in positions